The Pocket Diet
Perfect Portion Control that Works!

By George Kashou and
Caitlyn Lorenze, RD

A LINX Book

Acknowledgements

We would like to thank Community Memorial Hospital, Barb Taggart and her staff of dietitians, and all participants in the Pocket Diet study. We would also like to thank the many people who contributed their ideas during the development of this book.

The Pocket Diet

©2005 by George Kashou, Kangaroo Brands, Inc.
7620 North 81st Street, Milwaukee, WI 53223
Pocket Diet website: www.pocketdiet.com
All rights reserved. No part of this book may be reproduced
in any form without the prior written permission of the publisher.
ISBN: 0-9642386-9-1
Printed in the United States of America
Second Printing August 2005

Book design by Paul Fitzgerald
Contributing writing by Sandra Gurvis
Editing by Andrew Saunders

You should always consult with your doctor before making any changes to your diet, or starting an exercise program.

Table of Contents

FOREWORD: DONNA M. MANNING, DTR,   5
REGISTERED DIETETIC TECHNICIAN

INTRODUCTION
Why the Pocket Diet?   7
About the Pocket Diet Creators   8
About the Chef Who Developed the Recipes   9

CHAPTER 1: THE POCKET DIET:
AN EFFECTIVE WAY TO MANAGE YOUR WEIGHT
Obesity: An American Epidemic   10
What Is The Pocket Diet?   13
Pocket Diet Study: Proven Effective and Satisfying   14
Diet and Weight Loss Facts   16
In a Pita: The Basic Pocket Diet Plan   18
Convenience: The Pita Difference   19

CHAPTER 2: WEIGHT LOSS 101
Metabolism - Your Body's Engine   21
Does Dieting Work?   21
Body Mass Index: What You Should Weigh   22
Basal Metabolic Rate: How Much Should You Eat?   24
Changing and Dealing with Metabolism   25
Water, Water, Everywhere   26
Weight Loss Tips and Traps   27

CHAPTER 3: GOOD NUTRITION: YOU AND YOUR FOOD
Eating Healthy, Losing Weight   29
The New Food Pyramid   30
Nutrition Facts: What They Are, How to Read Labels   31
The Skinny on Fats   33

Cholesterol - The Good and the Bad   35
Proteins: The Body's Building Blocks   36
The Importance of Fiber   37
Sodium: Good, but in Moderation   38
Carbohydrates: The Staff of Life   39
Are Low-carb Diets Safe and Effective?   40

CHAPTER 4: FITNESS: A LIFETIME COMMITMENT

Introducing Exercise Into Your Life   43
Walking Is a Great Place to Start   44
Stretching, Aerobics, and Strength Training: Keeping It Balanced   46
Physical Activity and Calories Burned   48

CHAPTER 5: THE POCKET DIET MEAL PLAN

How Many Calories Do You Need?   51
Meals and the Pocket Diet   51
Basic Meal Plans   52
Three -Meal Plans   54
Managing Snacks   57
Planning Your Meals   59
Keys to Long-Term Weight Loss   60

CHAPTER 6: RECIPES

                                                            61

APPENDIXES

                                                            119

Forward:

DONNA M. MANNING, DTR,
REGISTERED DIETETIC TECHNICIAN

Congratulations on choosing the Pocket Diet. There are many aspects of life that we cannot change. However, you can control your weight and opt to live a healthy lifestyle. It is up to you!

People have different reasons for deciding to adopt healthy eating habits. Whether it's for weight loss, more energy, or to simply live a longer and better life, you'll need to work on certain behaviors and learn new ones.

There are some things you can do to help you succeed. First, set reasonable and obtainable goals. They can be both short and long-term but should be realistic, inspiring you and giving you incentive to stick with the program. Gradual small changes can add up to positive results. It takes time to change behaviors, but anything worth having is worth the effort. So believe in yourself and visualize achieving your goals.

Next, list all the reasons why you have chosen a healthier lifestyle. Some could be to lose weight, look better, live longer, buy new clothes, or whatever comes to mind.

Third, make a list of actions to accomplish your goal. These could be: follow the Pocket Diet plan, walk 20 minutes a day, drink plenty of water, and so on. Include physical activity in this plan. Choose activities you enjoy: walking, biking, dancing, gardening, swimming and so on. Vary your activity to keep it fun. Have some workout partners to keep you motivated. All activities, even taking the stairs instead of the elevator, will burn calories. Physical activity is not only good for your health, but it also raises your metabolism and self-esteem. It will make you feel good and help you keep your goals in focus.

Once you finish your list, type it up and place it on your refrigerator or your bathroom mirror. Read the list often and make notes of your progress. These actions will empower and motivate you.

Fad diets come and go, but the key elements to controlling your weight for the long term are:

1. Educating your self on proper nutrition.
2. Adopting new habits so you can eat healthy.

These are the most effective ways to control your weight for a lifetime.

I endorse the Pocket Diet because it promotes common sense eating with a variety of great tasting foods. It is convenient to follow, and this makes it sustainable over a long period of time. Perhaps best of all, it teaches portion control, which is key to reducing calories and weight.

Think of food as fuel for your body. How much fuel does your body need so you feel good? Eating healthy is not just about weight loss and maintenance, but also creating balance between calories eaten and calories burned. This is key to controlling your weight. The Pocket Diet will help you to control your portions, calories, and weight.

They say you are what you eat… so what are you now? And what do you want to be?

Eating is one of life's greatest pleasures, and all foods can fit into a healthy lifestyle. One of the exciting things in choosing to be healthy is making choices that are best for you. It is not one size fits all. Discover what works, and make it fun. Life is a journey and you can help create your own destiny and enjoy it more by making healthy choices.

Along with being a dietetic technician (DTR) registered with the American Dietetic Association, Donna M. Manning is a professional motivational speaker in the field of nutrition.

Introduction

The Pocket Diet is an effective and convenient plan that uses tasty and nutritious pita pocket bread to teach portion control to help you achieve a healthy weight. This book also provides complete but concise and easy-to-understand information about basic and sound nutrition. It will help you determine how much food to eat based on your body type, understand your metabolism, and empower you to improve your health and control your weight for life.

By simply adopting the basics of portion control taught by the Pocket Diet, excess weight will be shed slowly and permanently. The Pocket Diet is a "back to the basics" approach that will help avoid the up-and-down, yo-yo effect inherent so many of today's diet plans.

The Pocket Diet will provide you with a smooth transition from your current eating habits to an improved and healthier way of eating. It is convenient to follow and easy to maintain because you are allowed to eat everyday foods and snacks.

Remember that *portion control* is the key to successful weight control. Our pocket diet is the only diet plan that offers a convenient, healthy and edible food container -- a wholesome bread product -- that will help control meal portions. Dieting to lose weight is not just about what you eat, but how much. Choosing the right foods is vital to maintaining good health.

Why the Pocket Diet?

The healthcare community knows more than ever about what foods help the human body to be lean, energetic and efficient. More is being discovered each day about the links between obesity and heart disease, cancer, diabetes and other ailments. Yet the public is gaining weight at an alarming rate.

Losing weight has always been tough work. With current on-the-go lifestyles and dual income families, the days of spending long afternoons preparing meals with healthy, fresh foods from the garden and the butcher's are long gone. Family dinners have been replaced with a cell phone call checking in to see who is going to be picking what from which carryout. And the job of portion control has been turned over to restaurants and fast food chains.

There is a better way. With the Pocket Diet, you can eat deliciously and nutritiously in spite of today's fast-paced, fast-food lifestyles. This book offers simple and practical tips for lifelong portion control, weight loss, and healthy eating. Much of the information is based on the research from the National Institutes of Health, the American Heart Association, and the Institute of Medicine. But we've put it together so it's easy to follow and will work.

About the Pocket Diet Creators:

George Kashou

Of Mediterranean heritage, George Kashou grew up in a family that practiced good nutrition, long before the topic became mainstream. He, his wife and two adult daughters still dine on this healthy cuisine.

George's idea of exercise and relaxation are one in the same. He enjoys projects that require hard physical labor, such as landscaping and gardening. He maintains, tills and plants a large organic garden that helps to feed five families with plenty of leftovers for co-workers. His idea of recreational heaven on earth is downhill skiing.

A lifelong entrepreneur, George is quick to recognize opportunities and implement ideas. Twenty-five years ago he and his brother John started Kangaroo Brands, Inc. a small bakery. George and John set out to Americanize pita pockets, an ethnic specialty bread with limited distribution. Along with producing a high quality pita pocket that was easy to use, they received a federal patent for the "greatest innovation since sliced bread," a pre-opened pita pocket that is easy to fill without tearing. Today they sell their pita pocket breads -- the #1 brand in Deli – Bakery section in the U.S. -- in over 9,000 retail stores here and in Canada. George is the vice-president of sales and marketing for Kangaroo Brands.

But despite these accomplishments, George felt more needed to be done. He was disturbed by negative influence and lack of safety in fad diets. His believed that such diets preyed on too many people, including members of his extended family and friends. He recognized a need for a sensible approach to weight loss and decided write a book on nutrition. The result can be found in these pages.

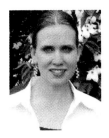

Caitlyn E. Lorenze, Registered Dietitian (RD)

A lifelong athlete, Caitlyn Lorenze has always understood the role of healthy eating and its relationship to optimal performance. From the field hockey grounds to the triathlon course, she has discovered firsthand how the right fuel can make the difference in achieving athletic and health goals.

This awareness and a passion for helping others improve their health through nutrition and fitness sparked her interest in nutrition at the academic level. Caitlyn earned a Bachelor's degree in Dietetics from the University of Maryland. Not losing sight on her link to athletics, Caitlyn also became a certified personal trainer, while simultaneously completing an internship with the American Dietetic Association at Virginia Polytechnic Institute and State University.

In 2003, Caitlyn founded wholesomebody, LLC to help individuals understand the role of nutrition in healthy living. The challenge of running a business, making healthy food choices and finding time for training has made Caitlyn truly appreciate the need for great-tasting, convenient good food, hence her participation in the Pocket Diet. Identifying simple ways to improve diet has become a trademark of her business.

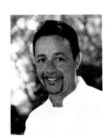

About the Chef Who Developed the Recipes

Scott Shully is a Milwaukee native and a well-known chef. He and his wife, Beth own Shully's Cuisine & Special Events. A graduate of Milwaukee Area Technical College's culinary arts programs, Scott was trained and certified at Societe Suisse des Hoteliers at Spa Hotel Bellevue in Braunwald, Switzerland.

His personal eating habits include a number of "mini" meals throughout the day. In designing the Pocket Diet program, he focused on quick and easy meal preparations, as well as a portion-controlled approach to eating healthy foods.

He believes in using fresh ingredients and tasty foods and is always trying out new and interesting ideas at work. But when cooking at home, he also sees the need for comfort, ease of preparation, and family enjoyment.

Because he wants eating to be a pleasure and not a chore, Scott's recipes cover a wide variety of healthy and nutritious foods that will help you lose weight.

"It has been my pleasure to assist in the development of the Pocket Diet's healthy, simple and tasty meals.

My personal eating habits include a number of "mini" meals throughout the day. I enjoyed the Pocket Diet's focus on quick and easy meal preparations, as well as its portion-controlled approach to eating healthy foods.

My approach to good eating is pretty straightforward: use fresh ingredients and foods you enjoy. At work, I am always trying new and interesting food ideas, but at home, comfort, ease of preparation and family enjoyment is essential.

Eating should be a pleasure, not a chore. You can enjoy a wide variety of healthy and nutritious foods – and still lose weight. This is the basic concept we have incorporated in the following recipes."

Obesity: An American Epidemic

At any given moment, approximately 50 million Americans are searching for the miracle diet -- some kind of fast, safe and easy way to lose weight and improve their health and outlook on life. There appears to be an ever-growing audience awaiting an instant panacea.

According to the Centers for Disease Control (www.cdc.gov) and the *Journal of the American Medical Association (JAMA):*

- Between the years 1960 and 2000 the number of obese adults in the US doubled.

- Currently 65% of Americans are overweight or obese, and this is a growing epidemic.

- $50 billion is spent annually on quackery diets, supplements and weight-loss devices.

The dieting dilemma is nothing new. "Diet consciousness" can be traced back to an 1869 book, "Letter on Corpulence," which was written by William Banting in London. The book sold for one shilling ($0.88), a miniscule trickle in what was to become a multi-billion dollar diet book industry.

Despite the thousands of diet books written since then, Americans still struggle to discover the Holy Grail of weight loss. As you will learn, the key to lifelong diet success is as simple as balance between sensible eating and maintaining an ongoing fitness program.

Chapter One

THE POCKET DIET: AN EFFECTIVE WAY TO MANAGE YOUR WEIGHT

What is The Pocket Diet?

The Pocket Diet offers a new twist to portion control:

- It is convenient, easy to follow and automatically teaches portion control through the use of a pita pocket "edible container" holding the right amount of a variety of healthy foods.

- It is based on eating and enjoying well-balanced meals from all food groups.

- It allows for two to three snacks per day.

- It benefits the entire family. There is no need to prepare special meals for those trying to lose weight.

- It offers easy, multiple-serving recipes that can be made in advance, refrigerated and then used as needed to prepare a quick meal.

Why The Pocket Diet was created

1. Many diets in today's marketplace are difficult to follow or make unrealistic demands on time-pressed consumers.

2. Pita pockets provide the ideal food container. One pocket bread holds the right portion size for a variety of healthy foods, and it fits the need of today's busy, on-the-go lifestyle.

3. Whole grain products are an integral part of a healthy and balanced diet. As such, learning to properly incorporate them into a weight loss plan can bring about great success.

4. Bread and complex carbohydrates are an important component of the food pyramid. Bread contains fiber, plant proteins, minerals and micronutrients. Carbohydrates are critical to proper brain function and are recommended as a supply of approximately 50% of the body's energy needs.

Pocket Diet Study: Proven Effective and Satisfying

The Pocket Diet was developed in cooperation with Community Memorial Hospital (CMH), in Menomonee Falls, Wisconsin. It was tested with a controlled study group of 38 participants during a six-week period.

Kangaroo Brands provided the recipes for breakfast, lunch and dinner. CMH dietitians analyzed the recipes for calories, fat, cholesterol, carbohydrates, sugars, protein and fiber. The flexible meal plans allowed the participants to select the recipe of their choice for any meal. Two meal plans were developed: a 1,500-calorie daily diet for people shorter than 5'6" and an 1,800-calorie for people taller than 5'6".

Participants were at least 15 pounds overweight, had a Body Mass Index (BMI) greater than 25 (BMI will be discussed in Chapter 2), and wanted to lose 1-2 pounds per week. They were weighed in weekly. Exercise was encouraged and alcohol consumption was discouraged. All 38 participants completed the study.

Results after six weeks:

- The group lost a total of 295 pounds
- The average weight loss was 8 pounds per person
- The greatest weight loss was 18 pounds; the least was 1.5 pounds
- The average weekly loss was 1.3 pounds per person
- The average pocket bread consumption was 4 pockets per day

**Follows are statements made by the participants
at the conclusion of the study:**

- "The pocket helped me control my meal portion"
- "The Pocket Diet was the easiest diet I have ever tried"
- "I was happy eating pocket bread on a daily basis"
- "The recipes were easy to prepare"
- "I have recommended this diet to my friends"

**A follow-up survey conducted 90 days after the study found
that of the 29 dieters who responded, (76% of the original 38)
found these results:**

- 79% of those surveyed were still following the Pocket Diet
- 73% had gotten closer to their weight loss objectives
- 94% were still using Kangaroo pocket breads as part of their daily diet

These findings suggest that the Pocket Diet is an effective way to lose weight and learn portion control. All of the participants were satisfied with the meal plan and the recipes provided and used the Kangaroo pocket breads to control their food portions. By following the USDA's food pyramid guidelines, the participants' nutritional needs were met as they lost weight.

Testimony: Barb Taggart, Registered Dietitian (RD)
Note: Ms. Taggart is the Supervisor of Clinical Dietetics at Community Memorial Hospital and she directed the diet study

Working on the Pocket Diet has been one of my most rewarding projects. It was truly amazing to watch the success of those who followed this program. It's really an instruction in healthy eating and portion control. Like most people, the participants were craving a program that taught them about good nutrition.

In this world of overabundance and fad diets, it has become difficult to know what normal eating really is. The Pocket Diet follows the basic principles of adequate amounts of carbohydrates, reduced fat and increased fiber. You develop a lifelong commitment to healthy eating when you get the right balance of nutrients including carbohydrates and protein. The Pocket Diet does that as well.

The results of the study spoke for themselves. All participants lost weight. They embraced the ability of the pocket bread to control their portions. Due to the convenience of the pocket bread, they utilized the plan while on vacation, caring for a sick parent or working full time. One participant, who had been told she would never lose weight due to her health condition, lost 14 pounds in 6 weeks! Perhaps best of all, most participants adopted the Pocket Diet as a way of life. As a registered dietitian, I am confident The Pocket Diet can help bring healthy eating back into focus for you!

Diet and Weight Loss Facts

But there's more to losing weight than following a diet. Dieting to lose weight is determined by how much you eat. Maintaining good health is all about the food you choose to eat. Sometimes these can be at cross-purposes.

Let's start by reviewing the process used to describe a safe, healthy and effective diet that will help you lose weight. Following are some facts about achieving and maintaining the proper weight and a healthy body:

1. You will gain weight if you consume more calories than your body burns off, and lose weight of you burn more calories than you consume.

2. 3,500 calories equals one pound of body weight. This means that if you consume 3,500 calories more than you burn, you will gain one pound. To lose one pound per week a person needs to burn 3,500 calories more per week than he or she consumes.

3. Exercise will increase your metabolism, help you burn calories and strengthen your heart.

4. Water is absolutely essential for health; drink a minimum of six, preferably eight, eight–ounce glasses per day.

5. Dietary fiber, found in natural foods such as whole grains, legumes, fruits and vegetables, is essential for a healthy intestinal tract and can help to improve cholesterol levels in some people.

6. Simple carbohydrates, such as the refined sugar found in convenience food, should be consumed sparingly, because they have little, if any, nutritional value. They only and provide "empty calories."

7. Complex carbohydrates are the body's preferred source of fuel for energy. They also provide fiber, which aids digestion.

8. Protein is essential for healthy body and muscle tissue. Meat, fish, legumes and dairy products are all excellent sources of protein.

9. Fats are essential. The healthiest fats are monounsaturated and polyunsaturated fats, which are found in seeds, nuts, fish oils and liquid vegetable oils. Saturated fats in meats and dairy should be consumed sparingly. Trans fats in solid shortenings, margarine, and many sweet baked goods, should be completely avoided.

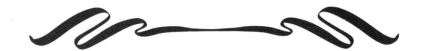

Quick Quiz

Ask Yourself the Following 15 Questions:

		YES	NO
1.	Do you eat different colored vegetables daily?	___	___
2.	Do you monitor your daily calorie intake?	___	___
3.	Do you cook more often than not?	___	___
4.	Do you often skip breakfast?	___	___
5.	Do you enjoy deep-fried foods?	___	___
6.	Do you like to eat a lot of food every day?	___	___
7.	Do you enjoy eating convenience food?	___	___
8.	Do you read the nutritional information on the foods you buy?	___	___
9.	Do you follow a regular exercise program?	___	___
10.	Do you frequent fast-food restaurants more than once per week?	___	___
11.	Do you eat bread?	___	___
12.	Do you know the difference between healthy and unhealthy foods?	___	___
13.	Do you know the nutritional value of foods you eat every day?	___	___
14.	Do you believe the expression, "You are what you eat"?	___	___
15.	Do you think will gain more weight by consuming your daily calories from carbs vs. protein and fat?	___	___

(Answers: 1. Y; 2. Y; 3.Y; 4.N; 5. N; 6. N; 7. N; 8.Y; 9.Y; 10.N; 11. Y; 12.Y; 13. Y; 14. Y; 15. N.) If you missed more than 5 questions, the following chapters will hopefully help you get them all right the next time you take the quiz.

Portion Control: An Essential Principle of The Pocket Diet

Most Americans struggle with their weight because they eat too much. The answer to maintaining proper weight is portion control. Because it's a 1.3-ounce, edible food container that holds hot or cold foods, the pita pocket will help you avoid eating too much.

Think of eating the same way as you would as managing your money. If you can manage a financial budget, then you can also learn to handle a caloric budget. First you need to know how many calories you can afford to consume, and second you need to learn the caloric values of foods. Always choose the best nutritional value for the foods selected, within your calorie limit.

In a Pita: The Basic Pocket Diet Plan

The plan is simple and described below. The key is to choose your foods carefully and get the best nutritional value for the calories you consume.

- Eat 3 meals per day using pita pockets to measure the portion size of your meals (You can choose almost any foods. Just make sure they fit into your pita pocket.)

- Eat 2-3 snacks per day (Designated portions of fruit, nuts, veggies, yogurt or cottage cheese)

- Slart and maintain an ongoing fitness program

Remember to ration the servings of the various foods throughout the day, to include three balanced meals plus 2-3 snacks in controlled portions.

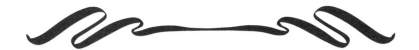

Pocket Diet Preview

The following illustrates the amount of food you will need to stay within approximately 1,500 calories per day. This sample menu provides a "taste" of what to expect in Chapter 5, which will have a thorough description of the meal plan.

Meal	*Food Choices*	*Approximate Calories*
Breakfast:	Egg, ham & cheese in 1 pocket	220
AM Snack:	Low-fat yogurt or fruit	100
Lunch:	Tuna or chicken salad in 2 pockets, and fruit	500
PM Snack:	Fruit, nuts, or raw veggies	130
Dinner:	4-5 oz. of meat or fish 1 serving complex carb + vegetable	450
Evening Snack	Fruit, nuts, yogurt or Reduced-fat ice cream	100
Total Calories		**1,500**

Convenience: The Pocket Diet Difference

One wonders why there are so many diets when the principles of safe and healthy weight loss are so basic. People are constantly seeking a "miracle" that will bring quick results without a lot of work.

A diet that requires significant effort may be difficult to sustain and ultimately lead to failure. We are creatures of habit. When asked to make sacrifices or otherwise drastically alter our habits, we rebel and ultimately fail.

That is why it is so important to be realistic when deciding on a diet, whether it is the Pocket Diet or another safe and realistic plan. Convenience is the key to success. Healthy, enjoyable and easy-to-prepare foods need to be available when you're hungry.

When considering a diet, ask yourself the following questions:

- Will my family and I enjoy eating the recommended foods?
- Are the foods easy to prepare?
- Does the diet require any significant extra work for my family and me?
- Is the diet safe and healthy?

Today's dual-income households and on-the-go lifestyles leave little time for meal preparation. The last thing you need is to spend more time and effort fixing special "diet" meals. Along with providing recipes, exercises, and nutrition tips, upcoming chapters will also help you manage your eating and make the best and most convenient choices for your lifestyle.

Chapter Two
WEIGHT LOSS 101

Metabolism - Your Body's Engine

Metabolism is your body's motor. It processes and burns calories. If your metabolism is idle, your body will burn only the minimum amount of calories necessary to keep the body functioning. However, even a slightly accelerated metabolic rate can be a significant help in burning extra calories.

Three critical elements accelerate or trigger your metabolism to burn calories.

1. *Exercise.* This is the best way to increase your metabolic rate. See chart on pages 48- 50 showing calories burned for various activity levels.

2. *Increase muscle mass.* Muscle burns calories. Even when you're inactive, it keeps your metabolism going at a higher rate.

3. *Proper eating.* When your body consumes food, it must process, or metabolize it. It's like fuel for your car. You must keep it filled up in order for it to run. But unlike your car, when your body is starved, your metabolism slows down to preserve its stored fuel, and therefore burns fewer calories per hour. Consequently, this metabolic slow down is why you should never skip meals. We recommend eating every 3-4 hours to keep your metabolism running at its most efficient speed.

Does Dieting Work?

Calories in food are derived from protein, carbohydrates and fat. Most of the 300+ diets in today's marketplace follow one of the basic principles listed below and are:

• Low in (saturated) fat for heart problems and reducing cholesterol

• Low glycemic for diabetes (restricting simple sugars or carbohydrates)

• Well-balanced/calorie measured

The Pocket Diet is a well-balanced, calorie-measured diet that follows the new USDA's food pyramid guide. The fiber in whole wheat and whole grain pita pockets contributes to a lower glycemic index compared to many foods. Low-fat fillings help maintain a heart- healthy approach.

Additionally, there are two types of diets:

- *Exclusive diets* that achieve weight loss by severely restricting what a person eats

- *Inclusive diets* that offer flexibility and choice, and focus on portion size and nutrition

The Pocket Diet is an inclusive diet. Rather than restricting what you eat, it guides you as to how much you should consume. The food choices are yours to make.

We hope you would choose the healthier foods, because you are what you eat. However, even if you indulge in some less-nutritious "favorites," the portion-control aspect of this diet will still help you lose weight.

Before beginning, you might want to ask yourself: "Am I dieting just to lose weight, or to improve my health?" Hopefully, your answer will be that you're dieting to improve your health – and lose weight in the process.

Body Mass Index: What You Should Weigh

Being overweight can aggravate arthritis or lower back problems and cause diabetes, heart disease and gallbladder disease. Excess weight has also been associated with breast, uterine, ovarian and other cancers. The government has developed a tool to determine your risk based on your weight called the Body Mass Index (BMI). Use the table below to determine your individual risk.

Calculating BMI is simple, quick, and inexpensive — but it does have limitations. One problem with using BMI as a measurement tool is that muscular or large boned people may fall into the "overweight" category when they are actually healthy and fit. Another problem with using BMI is that people who have lost muscle mass, such as the elderly, may be in the "healthy weight" category — according to their BMI — when they actually have reduced nutritional reserves. BMI, therefore, is useful as a general guideline to monitor trends in the population, but by itself is not diagnostic of an individual's health status. Further evaluation should be performed to determine associated health risks.

Body Mass Index Table

To use the table, find the appropriate height in the left-hand column labeled Height. Move across to a given weight. The number at the top of the column is the BMI at that height and weight. Pounds have been rounded off.

BMI	19	20	21	22	23	24	25	26	27	28	29	30	31	32	33	34	35	36	37	38	39	40
Height (Inches)																						
58	91	96	100	105	110	115	119	124	129	134	138	143	148	153	158	162	167	172	177	181	186	191
59	94	99	104	109	114	119	124	128	133	138	143	148	153	158	163	168	173	178	183	188	193	198
60	97	102	107	112	118	123	128	133	138	143	148	153	158	163	168	174	179	184	189	194	199	204
61	100	106	111	116	122	127	132	137	143	148	153	158	164	169	174	180	185	190	195	201	206	211
62	104	109	115	120	126	131	136	142	147	153	158	164	169	175	180	186	191	196	202	207	213	218
63	107	113	118	124	130	135	141	146	152	158	163	169	175	180	186	191	197	203	208	214	220	225
64	110	116	122	128	134	140	145	151	157	163	169	174	180	186	192	197	204	209	215	221	227	232
65	114	120	126	132	138	144	150	156	162	168	174	180	186	192	198	204	210	216	222	228	234	240
66	118	124	130	136	142	148	155	161	167	173	179	186	192	198	204	210	216	223	229	235	241	247
67	121	127	134	140	146	153	159	166	172	178	185	191	198	204	211	217	223	230	236	242	249	255
68	125	131	138	144	151	158	164	171	177	184	190	197	204	210	216	223	230	236	243	249	256	262
69	128	135	142	149	155	162	169	176	182	189	196	203	210	216	223	230	236	243	250	257	263	270
70	132	139	146	153	160	167	174	181	188	195	202	209	216	222	229	236	243	250	257	264	271	278
71	136	143	150	157	165	172	179	186	193	200	208	215	222	229	236	243	250	257	265	272	279	286
72	140	147	154	162	169	177	184	191	199	206	213	221	228	235	242	250	258	265	272	279	287	294
73	144	151	159	166	174	182	189	197	204	212	219	227	235	242	250	257	265	272	280	288	295	302
74	148	155	163	171	179	186	194	202	210	218	225	233	241	249	256	264	272	280	287	295	303	311
75	152	160	168	176	184	192	200	208	216	224	232	240	248	256	264	272	279	287	295	303	311	319
76	156	164	172	180	189	197	205	213	221	230	238	246	254	263	271	279	287	295	304	312	320	328

Weight (Pounds)

A healthy weight is an index of 19-25, moderately overweight is an index of 26-29, and severely overweight is an index over 30.

Keep in mind this BMI chart does not take into consideration an individual's bone structure or muscle mass. People that are large boned or have more muscle mass may weigh more than this chart shows, but still be in a healthy weight range.

Basal Metabolic Rate: How Much Should You Eat

The answer depends on your current weight, activity level, age, and metabolism, but eating is only one part of the formula.

A sedentary woman burns only 10 calories per pound of body weight (A man burns 11 calories). That means a 150-pound female would burn 1,500 calories per day just to keep her heart beating, lungs breathing and brain functioning. The minimum number of calories your body requires to maintain itself if you were laying down all day and night in a sedentary position (but not sleeping) is referred to as the body's Basal Metabolic Rate (BMR).

Calories burned increase dramatically with physical activity. This is referred to as the AMR, or the Active Metabolic Rate. This determines the number of calories your body burns for its activity level. For example, a lightly active, 150-pound female may burn off 1800 calories per day.

The following information will help you calculate the number of calories you burn in a normal day. In this way, you can determine how many calories you can consume and still lose weight. However, once the weight is lost you should continue being active. In order to maintain your desired weight, you must continually balance your daily intake with your level of activity and the calories your body burns.

Still, we all overeat occasionally. What's important is to make a conscious effort to balance any over-consumption with extra activity, or to reduce consumption on subsequent days.

Calorie Chart

Formula: Weight X Multiplier = Calories burned per day
(i.e., The BMR for a woman is: 10 X 150lb. = 1,500 calories
The BMR for a man : 11 X 200 lb. = 2,200 calories)

Activity Level	Woman (multiplier)	Men (multiplier)
BMR- Sedentary:	10	11
Light Activity:	12	13
Moderate Exercise:	13	14
Moderate/Heavy Exercise:	15	16
Regular Heavy Exercise	17	18

For example, a 200-pound man who is sedentary burns 2,200 calories per day (200 x 11). The same man with moderate exercise burns 2,800 calories per day (200 x 14). An average 150 lb. woman who is sedentary burns 1,500 calories per day (150 x 10). With moderate exercise she burns 1,950 calories (150 x 13).

A woman with moderate exercise alone burns an extra 18,000 calories per month. This translates into a weight loss of 5 pounds or 1.25 pounds per week. (600 x 30 days =18,000 divided by 3500 calories per pound = 5 lbs.).

Changing and Dealing with Metabolism

Metabolism is the process that converts food to energy. Think of metabolism as the speed at which your body's engine operates. Basal metabolism is the energy you need when your body's engine is idling – when you're in a reclined position. It gives your body the energy it needs to maintain its basic functions and accounts for about 75% of the calories expended daily.

Some people have faster body engines. Because their basal metabolism is higher, they burn off more calories. People with a lower basal metabolism will have a more difficult time burning off calories.

The good news is that there are safe methods to improve your metabolic rate.

Eight Safe and Natural Ways To Rev Up Your Metabolism

1. Always eat breakfast. Skipping breakfast puts the body in a defensive mode. When the body senses it is low on fuel (food), it slows your metabolic rate to conserve energy.

2. Never eat less than 1,200 calories per day. Your body needs a minimum of 1,200 calories daily just to perform its basic functions. Anything less will prompt the body to slow down its processes, including metabolism.

3. Snack on complex carbohydrates. Fruits, vegetables, and grains fuel your metabolism, and have fewer calories per gram than fat (Carbs have 4 calories per gram vs. the 9 calories per gram in fats).

4. Exercise on a daily basis. Daily exercise will improve your metabolism. A brisk 15-30 minute walk after lunch or dinner energizes the body by boosting your heart rate and blood flow.

5. Tone your muscles with weight training. Toned muscles charge your metabolism and muscle naturally burns more calories.

6. Avoid alcohol. Alcohol depresses your metabolism while stimulating appetite.

7. Look for situations to be active. Instead of finding the closest parking spot, park farther away and walk the distance. Use stairs instead of elevators. These small things can significantly increase the amount of exercise you get each day.

8. Stay hydrated. Try to drink a cup of water every few hours, drinking eight or more 8-oz glasses a day. Your body needs plenty of water to function optimally. Carry a bottle of water with you and drink throughout the day.

Water, Water, Everywhere

Water, the most common substance on earth, is also the nutrient that your body needs the most. Between 60-70% of an adult's body weight is water. Water is critical in regulating all organs and body temperature, as well as dissolving solids and carrying nutrients throughout the body.

Dehydration is the loss of water and electrolytes needed for normal body functioning. Staying hydrated is essential to keeping yourself healthy.

Symptoms of dehydration include:

- Lightheadedness, dizziness, headaches and nausea
- Muscle fatigue, cramps and a general loss of endurance
- Fainting, in cases of extreme dehydration

Severe dehydration can lower blood pressure, weaken the heart, and shut down the kidneys. One of the best ways to recognize dehydration is to pay close attention to the color of your urine. Ideally, light to clear urine indicates proper water intake. Dark yellow urine may be a sign of dehydration.

The average person should drink 8 eight-ounce glasses of water or other fluids daily. Do not substitute coffee, tea or soda for water. Caffeine in particular acts as a diuretic, pulling water from your body.

Tips For Keeping Yourself Hydrated:

- Drink extra water on hot summer days, or if you stay outdoors for extended periods of time in cold weather. Dehydration occurs more rapidly in extreme temperatures through perspiration and breathing.

- Caffeine, alcohol and tobacco dehydrate the body. Drink equal amounts of water to equal your consumption of alcohol or caffeine.

Weight Loss Tips and Traps

Choosing a weight loss program is almost as important as selecting a career. It can greatly improve your quality of life (or conversely have a negative impact on your health), so evaluate each diet carefully. Weight loss depends on controlling the calories consumed, regular exercise, curtailing convenience food and making a long-term commitment to healthy eating habits.

Follows are five tips for long-term success:

1. Never skip breakfast. Eating breakfast charges your metabolism and gives your body the energy it needs to get through the morning.

2. Drink eight 8-oz. glasses of water or fluids every day.

3. Eat like your ancestors. Your diet should include fruits, vegetables, grains & breads, legumes, lean meats and fish. Avoid convenience and highly processed foods.

4. Eat something nutritious every three to four hours.

5. Stay physically active.

On the other hand, avoid such weight loss "traps" as:

- You can eat as many low-fat foods as you desire. (Zero grams of fat does not equal zero calories)

- There are different kinds of calories. (A calorie is a calorie)

- It is possible to lose 50 pounds in 6 weeks, 5 pounds in a weekend, or any number of pounds without exercise. (It is possible, but not healthy. Rapid weight loss is mostly water weight and this can result in dehydration, which is very dangerous.)

- You can shed pounds by merely wearing a belt, ring or bracelet. (Yes, and the Brooklyn Bridge is for sale, too!)

Also be very careful with drugs that claim to aid in weight loss. They may have dangerous side effects that may not be immediately noticeable.

Follows are some examples of how diets can be easily sabotaged.

- One extra meal at fast food restaurant contains approximately 1500 calories: 700 calories in the sandwich, 540 calories in the French fries and 310 calories in the drink. Add a shake for dessert and you're up to 2,000 calories in just one meal!

- Three slices of pizza and a large soft drink will add about 1,200 calories to your diet.

- Ten crème sandwich cookies will cost you 550 calories, or one-fourth of your recommended daily caloric intake.

- Beware of snacking. Potato chips, cookies, donuts and candy bars are all convenience foods that are easily consumed in large quantities. Even peanuts, which are healthy, are high in calories. A snack can easily add up to an extra 500 calories without your realizing it.

Be aware of the nutritional and caloric content of the foods you consume. As you can see, it's easy to hit 4,000 to 5,000 calories in a day. And it only takes 3,500 excess calories to create one new pound of fat on your body.

Chapter Three

GOOD NUTRITION: YOU AND YOUR FOOD

Eating Healthy, Losing Weight

Your weight will ultimately be determined by calories consumed versus calories burned. A calorie is still a calorie, whether it is derived from fat, protein or carbohydrates. Calories are all equal in adding or decreasing body weight. All diets, including low-carb diets, can only be effective for long-term weight loss by limiting calories. The key to long-term weight loss is finding a convenient way to achieve a healthy balance of carbohydrates, protein and fat while maintaining an appropriate caloric intake.

Weight loss diets offer the reader many different approaches to manage the calories consumed. Some diets simply go too far with empty promises that take advantage of people's vulnerabilities.

If there is a "magic bullet" to controlling your weight it would be in your ability to control your portions and learning the caloric value of the foods you eat. How healthy you are is often a result of the nutritional content of the foods you choose to eat.

The Pocket Diet is a sustainable and healthy way to eat a variety of good food. When combined with an exercise regimen, it will help you achieve and maintain your desired weight and improve your overall health.

Remember, the most sustainable and safest way to lose weight is by reducing caloric intake to a level slightly lower than what your body burns through normal activity. Combine this with the consumption of well-balanced meals that include healthy food choices, and adopt a reasonable exercise regimen you can enjoy and sustain.

Start with a commitment to yourself to adopt and practice what you have learned in this book. Stay focused on that commitment, and the rewards of achieving a healthier weight and lifestyle will be inevitable. Your mind and body will need time to be redirected. You can achieve your goals if you are patient, forgiving and tenacious in your effort.

The New Food Pyramid

The U.S. Department of Agriculture (USDA) updated the U.S. Food Guide Pyramid in early 2005. When the old pyramid was developed in 1992, there was a lot less knowledge about and emphasis on whole grain foods than there is today. Also the link between exercise and staying healthy was not fully taken into consideration.

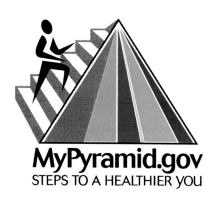

MyPyramid.gov
STEPS TO A HEALTHIER YOU

The new food pyramid is designed to provide a general guideline to healthy eating. Unlike the old pyramid, which showed only foods, it has been updated to include physical activity. The drawing of a person climbing stairs at the side of the new pyramid is a reminder that physical activity is as important to healthy living as eating well.

Food groups are illustrated as a series of differently sized colored bands. The colors are:
– Orange for grains
– Green for vegetables
– Red for fruit
– Yellow for fats and oils
– Blue for dairy
– Purple for meats, beans, and fish

The bands are different widths to show how much of a particular food group a person should eat each day. So the orange band is wider than the yellow one because people need to eat more grains than fats and oils.

The pyramid also emphasizes the following points:

- *Combine exercise with eating well.* Food and exercise are closely linked. Exercise benefits every part of the body, including the mind. Experts now know that exercise fights off a range of possible health problems like heart disease, diabetes, and even depression. It is now recommended that people should strive to 60 minutes of moderate to vigorous exercise every day. This may be a challenge, but start small and try to work up to one hour over time.

- *Eat a variety of foods.* The different color bands in the pyramid send the message that it's important to eat lots of different foods. Not only does it provide people with a good balance of nutrients, but the variety of tastes helps develop an affinity for healthy foods.

Nutrition Facts: What They Are, How to Read Labels

Food labels—usually called Nutrition Facts—are valuable in making healthy eating an essential part of everyday meal planning. Most foods found in grocery stores today list their particular Nutrition Facts on a label typically located on the back or side of their package. Reading a food label is simple when you know what to look for.

Select your grocery items according to the following rules:

1. Is it a reasonable serving size? A good gauge is how many servings you could eat at one sitting.

2. Choose foods that are generally low in fat and high in fiber. Foods with less salt and less sugar, and those made with whole-grain ingredients are your best selections.

Nutrition Facts

Serving Size (30g)
Servings Per Container

Amount Per Serving

Calories 80   Calories from Fat 0

	% Daily Value*
Total Fat 0g	0%
Saturated Fat 0g	0%
Cholesterol 0mg	0%
Sodium 160mg	7%
Total Carbohydrate 17g	6%
Dietary Fiber less than 1 gram	3%
Sugars 0g	
Protein 3g	

Vitamin A 0%	•	Vitamin C 0%	
Calcium 2%	•	Iron 4%	

*Percent Daily Values are based on a 2,000 calorie diet. Your daily values may be higher or lower depending on your calorie needs:

	Calories:	2,000	2,500
Total Fat	Less than	65g	80g
Saturated Fat	Less than	20g	25g
Cholesterol	Less than	300mg	300mg
Sodium	Less than	2,400mg	2,400mg
Total Carbohydrate		300g	375g
Dietary Fiber		25g	30g

Calories per gram:
Fat 9 • Carbohydrate 4 • Protein 4

Serving Size

This is the most important piece of information on the label. It tells you how many servings are in the container. If one serving is one cookie, for example, and you eat three cookies, make sure you calculate the rest of the information on three servings.

Calories

How many calories are there per serving? Multiply the amount of calories by how many servings you actually had.

Sodium

Packaged foods are generally high in sodium. If you are on a sodium-restricted diet, choose foods that contain 140 milligrams or less of sodium per serving; aim for less than a total of 2,400 milligrams of sodium per day.

Fat

Not all fat is bad. In fact, fat is essential for hormone function and vitamin and mineral transport...and fat makes food taste good! However, not all fats are healthy fats; saturated fat and trans-fats may contribute to heart disease. And fat has more than double the calories of protein and carbohydrates, therefore a smaller volume of high-at foods contains more fat than a larger volume of low fat foods. So pay close attention to the fat content on food labels.

Carbohydrates, Sugar and Fiber

The total number of carbohydrates is reported on the nutrition facts panel along with the amount of sugar and fiber contained in one serving. Sugar is the simplest form of carbohydrate, and in the body all carbohydrate is broken down into sugar, or "glucose." Use the Nutrition Facts label to learn how many grams of sugar a product contains.

Also, when reviewing the ingredients in a food, look for foods that do not list sugar in the first three ingredients. Sugar may be listed under a number of names such as, brown sugar, dextrose, fructose, glucose, high fructose corn syrup, lactose, maltose, malt syrup, raw sugar, sucrose, and syrup. For example, when comparing breakfast cereals, choose the brand that contains the least amount of added sugar and most fiber.

Fiber helps the human body with a number of tasks, including aiding in normal bowel function, promoting regularity, and controlling blood sugar levels. It also reduces risk of colon cancer and lowers blood cholesterol. To reach the recommended fiber intake of 25-35 grams per day, look for foods that contain at least 3 grams of fiber.

The Skinny on Fats

Fats occur naturally in food and are added to food products. They play an important role in nutrition by providing a concentrated source of energy for the body.

The body uses fat to store energy, insulate body tissue, and transport fat-soluble vitamins through the blood. Fats also enhance the flavor of food and make baked products tender.

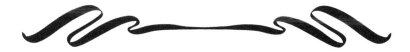

The Good, Not-So-Good, and Really Dangerous
Not all fats are created equal. There are four types:

1. Monounsaturated Fats (Good) are liquid at room temperature, but become solid when refrigerated. Examples of these fats include olive oil and canola oil. Monounsaturated fats may help improve cholesterol levels if used to replace saturated fats in the diet.

2. Polyunsaturated Fats (Good) remain liquid even while refrigerated. One type of polyunsaturated fat is worth special note:

   Omega - 3 fatty acids (Good) are special fats essential for normal body function, they are important components of cell membranes throughout the body, especially the eyes, brain and sperm cells. These fats regulate blood clotting, contraction and relaxation of the artery walls and inflammation. They have been shown to have significant benefits in the prevention of heart disease and stroke. The best sources of Omega-3s are fatty fish (like salmon), walnuts, flaxseed, and canola and soybean oil.

3. Saturated Fats (Bad) are solid at room temperature and include beef fat, butter, etc. These fats are typically found in animals and some plants and may increase bad cholesterol (LDL).

4. Trans-Fats (Bad) are artificially made through the hydrogenation of unsaturated fats that have fats. They are found in certain processed foods, they may raise bad cholesterol (LDL) and lower good cholesterol (HDL).

The amount of fat eaten is as important as the types of fat consumed. Food fats consist of units called fatty acids that raise or lower blood cholesterol. Eat all types of fat in moderation, because fats contain more than twice the calories of proteins or carbohydrates.

The American Heart Association recommends keeping calories from fat at 25-35% of total calories consumed and saturated fats at less then 10% of total calories. For example, if you are consuming a diet of 1500 calories

Total Fat:

> 1500 calories x 30% = 450 calories from fat
> 450 calories from fat / 9 calories per gram = 50 grams of total fat per day

Saturated Fat:

> 1500 calories x 10% = 150 calories from saturated fat
> 150 calories from saturated fat / 9 calories per gram = 16 grams of saturated fat per day

The Danger of Trans-fats

Nevertheless, trans-fats should be avoided altogether. They are formed by the partial hydrogenation of vegetable oil, a chemical process that alters its nutrients. Hydrogenation solidifies oil to make it resemble real foods, such as butter. It is used to add texture to food products and to increase their shelf life.

Trans-fats have no nutritional value. In fact, studies show that trans-fats can be detrimental to your health. As a result, beginning in January 2006 the FDA requires manufacturers to list all trans-fats on nutritional labels.

Daily Fat Intake Guide - 1 gram of fat = 9 calories

Calorie Level	Total Fat Grams	Saturated Fat Grams	Reduced Fat Diet	
			Total Fat Grams	Saturated Fat Grams
1,500	45	15	33	10
1,800	55	18	40	13
2,000	60	20	45	14
2,200	66	22	50	16

Type of Fatty Acid	Effect on Cholesterol	Found In	Daily Usage
Monounsaturated	Lowers bad, Raises good	Avocados, peanuts, peanut oil, canola oil and olive oil.	10 to 15% of total calories
Polyunsaturated	Lowers bad	Vegetable oils (safflower, sunflower, corn), sunflower seeds. Main fats in seafood.	10% of total calories
Saturated	Raises bad	Animal fat, (butter, whole milk, ice cream, meat, poultry skin) coconut and palm oil.	Less than 10% of total calories
Trans	Raises bad, Lowers good	Hydrogenated vegetable fats (shortening, margarine), fried foods, baked goods, snacks.	Avoid

Cholesterol - The Good and the Bad

Every person's blood has cholesterol. Cholesterol helps produce cell membranes and hormones and serves other important functions. The body generates all of the cholesterol it needs; however, additional cholesterol may be derived from the consumption of meats, eggs, fish, poultry, cheese, milk and other animal products. In addition, some foods may trigger the body to produce extra cholesterol. These include products containing trans-fats and saturated fats.

If the cholesterol content of the blood stream gets too high, cholesterol particles begin sticking to the walls of the blood vessels and arteries, slowly narrowing the passageway and restricting blood flow. This condition is called arteriosclerosis, and a symptom of heart disease. Over 100 million American have total cholesterol of 200 mg/dl or higher and either have developed or are at risk for developing cardiovascular disease.

Maintaining normal cholesterol levels (less than 200 mg/dl) is a proven way to prevent cardiovascular disease. Eating foods low in saturated fat and cholesterol and avoiding trans-fats will help with this, as will physical exercise. Also, visit your doctor every 1-2 years, especially if you're over 40, to determine if your levels of total cholesterol, HDL and LDL are in a safe range.

Good vs. Bad Cholesterol

In addition to maintaining an overall cholesterol level of 200 mg/dl or less, it is also important to know how much of your cholesterol is "good" and how much is "bad."

Cholesterol and other fats do not dissolve in blood and have to be transported to cells in your body with carriers called lipoproteins. There are two types of lipoproteins:

- High-Density Lipoproteins (HDL) which carry cholesterol away from the arteries and back to the liver where they are cleansed from the body. HDL is the "good" (or Healthy) cholesterol.

- Low-density lipoproteins (LDL) may deposit cholesterol and other substances on artery walls, causing the artery to narrow. LDL is the "bad" (or Lousy) cholesterol. Saturated fats and trans-fats contribute to increases in LDL levels.

You can raise your good (HDL) cholesterol by exercising, not smoking and staying at a healthy weight.

Proteins: The Body's Building Blocks

Protein and fat are the building materials of the body. Proteins are everywhere in the body – in our muscles, organs, tissue, bones, brain cells, blood cells, genetic matter, skin, hair and fingernails, etc.

Protein is essential for healthy living because it supports the constant repair and renewal that takes place inside our bodies.

Because the body cannot store protein, it must be replenished daily. The best protein sources are egg whites, legumes (beans), soy products, grains, poultry, fish and low-fat dairy products because they are low in fat and cholesterol.

Benefits of soy protein

Soy products have been a standard part of the diet in China, Japan, Indonesia, and other Asian countries for centuries. In these countries, it is believed that soy products can help prevent disease.

Modern research is showing that small to moderate intake of soy has many healthy benefits:

- It is a good source of low-fat protein

- It may prevent osteoporosis and heart disease

- It may help prevent colon, breast, uterus and prostate cancer

- If can be a rich source of calcium, iron, zinc, phosphorus, magnesium, B vitamins, omega-3 fatty acids and fiber. However not all soy products have equal amounts of these nutrients.

The Important of Fiber

Many health experts advise people of all ages to consume more dietary fiber. There is considerable research suggesting that a diet with 25-35 grams of daily fiber may reduce the incidence of diabetes, heart disease, colon cancer and obesity.

Even though fiber is one of the most important components of a healthy diet, most Americans consume less than half the daily requirement. Fiber has no calories because the body cannot absorb it; however, it is essential for healthy bowel movements.

Insufficient dietary fiber is the usual cause of chronic constipation. This can lead to a myriad of other health problems such as hemorrhoids and varicose veins, which result from excessive straining when passing a stool. It is normal to have 1-2 easily passed bowel movements a day.

The American Dietetic Association recommends the following daily fiber consumption:

- Adults: 25-35 grams

- Children: Their age plus 5-10 grams each day

There are two types of dietary fiber: soluble and insoluble. *Insoluble* fiber passes through your digestive tract largely intact. It provides the bulk needed for proper stool formation. Insoluble fiber is found in most fruits, vegetables, whole-wheat breads, grains, wheat and corn bran, whole grains, and legumes. Adequate amounts of liquid are needed for this fiber to be effective.

Soluble fiber, which forms a gel when mixed with liquid, works in conjunction with insoluble fiber by helping to form the stool. Soluble fiber may also lower cholesterol by removing bile acids that digest saturated fat. Soluble fiber can also slow the absorption of sugars after a meal, thus reducing the amount of insulin the pancreas must produce. Stabilizing insulin levels reduces the stress on the pancreas. Soluble fiber is found in many fruits and vegetables, oat bran, oatmeal, barley and beans.

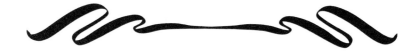

Simple Ways to Incorporate Fiber

- Add bran to muffins, pancake batter, casseroles, breakfast cereals, salads and yogurt.

- Boost the fiber content in cereals with fresh fruit and a sprinkling of bran.

- Choose whole-grain baked goods with raisins or other dried fruits.

Sodium: Good, but in Moderation

Salt contains sodium, an essential mineral for maintaining life. It controls our body's ability to retain water and maintains the critical balance between cells and body fluids. It also aids in the contraction of muscle tissue and serves as a vital ingredient in blood plasma and digestive secretions.

Excessive salt intake, however, may aggravate high blood pressure, hypertension and cardiovascular problems.

The National Academy of Sciences recommends that Americans consume a minimum of 500 mg of sodium per day to maintain normal body functions. Consuming up to 2,500 mg per day is still considered safe.

Unfortunately, the sodium intake of most Americans averages closer to 5,000-7,000 mg per day, most of it coming from processed and ready-made foods.

Ways to Reduce Salt Intake:

- Cook from scratch. Reduce the consumption of prepared foods containing large amounts of sodium
- Instead of using salt, squeeze fresh lemon juice on steamed vegetables, broiled fish, rice or pasta for a refreshing taste
- Season your food with fresh herbs, wines, peppers and alternate spices, as well as with vegetable and citrus juice
- Choose fresh, frozen or canned vegetables that don't have added salt
- Snack on fresh fruits and vegetables, which are naturally low in sodium
- Enjoy salty snacks in moderation.

Carbohydrates: The Staff of Life

Carbohydrates have become a hot topic of debate ever since the introduction of the high-protein diet, which advocates a dramatic reduction in carbohydrate intake to reduce weight. However, carbohydrates help the body perform vital functions:

- They are the primary source of the body's energy
- They have a protein-sparing effect that protects muscle tissue from breaking down
- They are the primary fuel source for the brain
- They provide many important nutrients, including dietary fiber, which is essential for the digestive track.

Carbohydrates can be complex or simple. Complex carbohydrates are good because they contain cellulose/fiber, are very important for digestion and may also help prevent colon cancer. Most Americans consume less than half of the recommended daily amount of dietary fiber, which should be approximately 30 grams per day.

Complex carbohydrates are found in foods such as:

- Bread, pasta, rice and potatoes
- Whole-grain products
- Legumes (dried beans)
- Fruits & vegetables

Most Simple carbohydrates are empty calorie foods, which means they add calories without doing anything beneficial for the body. As a result, they should be consumed sparingly. Simple carbohydrates are found in candy, cookies, cakes, sodas, sugar-added juices and other products that contain refined sugar. However, some foods like fruits contain both simple and complex carbohydrates, such as natural sugars, fiber and other nutrients.

Are Low-Carb Diets Safe and Effective

The past decade has seen a great deal of controversy over the safety and efficacy of low-carb diets. This craze has left many people confused as to which foods are healthy. Still, there are some facts that most dietitians, doctors and health associations agree on:

- A healthy diet is high in fiber and low in saturated fat.
- Losing body fat and maintaining a healthy weight require sustainable healthy food choices.
- Low-carb diets for many are unrealistic on a long-term basis.
- Consuming too many calories, in the form of protein, fat, carbohydrate, or alcohol will result in weight gain.

The restriction of bread products in low-carb diets is neither valid nor healthy. Breads are an important source of complex carbohydrates and play a vital role in overall body function. They should not be confused with simple carbohydrates, the empty calories of refined sugars found in candy, soda and ordinary convenience food. People of all cultures have enjoyed bread for thousands of years.

> *"Americans have been so bombarded with information about low-carb diets that they incorrectly perceive bread to be a "bad" food, whereas bread is one of the healthiest and most nutrient-rich carbohydrates. Cutting bread from your diet is not the answer for people concerned about their long-term health."*
>
> *-- Carolyn O'Neil, Registered Dietitian (RD) and Former CNN nutrition correspondent*

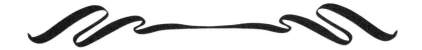

Pita Pockets and Carbohydrates
The question is: "Can you lose weight by reducing your carb intake?"

The answer is: Yes, but you needn't reduce carb intake so drastically that you put your health in jeopardy. Eliminating simple carbohydrates (convenience food), while reducing total carbohydrates, in proportion to an appropriate reduction in daily calories, should bring about successful and maintainable weight loss.

For example, a 1-ounce slice of sandwich bread contains approximately 15 grams of carbohydrates and 60 calories. A sandwich made with two slices of bread would have 120 calories or 30 grams of carbohydrates.

A 1.3-ounce Kangaroo wheat pocket, which is all you need to make a sandwich, contains only 80 calories and 16 grams of carbohydrates. The Kangaroo Pocket reduces the total calories from each sandwich by 40 calories and 14 grams of carbohydrates.

Chapter Four

FITNESS: A LIFETIME COMMITMENT

Introducing Exercise Into Your Life

Nutrition and fitness experts agree that if you want to lose weight faster and keep it off you need to start and maintain an ongoing fitness program. This can be accomplished with only 30 minutes of activity per day. Every motion your body makes burns calories. The more you move, the more you lose!

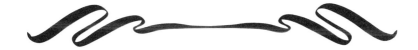

Fitness Facts

- Even something as simple as a brisk, two-block walk every day can help you lose 10 pounds a year!

- Living healthfully is living happily. Exercise releases your brain's endorphins, powerful, naturally produced analgesics that make you feel better.

- Regular exercise is a great way to reduce stress. Research shows that headaches, chronic pain and other common physical conditions are aggravated by everyday stress. A 15-minute walk is a natural way to promote health–and, best of all, it's free.

One sure way to insure fitness success is to make it fun. Follows are some suggestions in finding an activity that will hopefully become a lifelong habit.

1. *Do what you like.* Because physical activity is only effective when you actually do it, choose something you enjoy. If running bores you, don't run. Go for a bike ride, try a new aerobics or boxing class. Keep trying new ways to get active until you find something you enjoy.

2. *Start slow.* If you are new to exercise or have not exercised in a while, begin slowly, such as with a walking program.

3. *Don't do it alone.* Exercise with a friend, family member or co-worker. A partner increases enjoyment, decreases boredom and helps to keep you motivated.

4. *Be flexible, but make it a priority.* Do what and when you can, but make sure exercise is a part of your schedule.

5. *Listen to music.* Music helps time pass quickly. It also will improve your endurance and tolerance for repetitive physical activity.

6. *Add variety to your fitness routine.* Choose more than one type of physical activity. This not only prevents boredom but works different muscle groups. Select an indoor and an outdoor activity to allow for changes in the weather or your schedule.

If you are uncertain what to do or where to start, you seek advice from a trainer or other fitness professional.

Walking is a Great Place to Start

One of the most convenient and low-risk ways to get started with a fitness program is by walking. A regular walking program can help reduce blood cholesterol, lower blood pressure, increase cardiovascular endurance, boost bone strength, burn calories, and keep weight down.

Walking Tips

1. Start out slowly. Going too far or too fast too soon is the number one cause of injuries. Start with a comfortable distance and then try to add five minutes each week until you reach 60 minutes.

2. Intermittent sessions are just as effective as continuous ones. If your health or schedule does not permit a 20- to 60-minute session of walking, break your sessions down into 10- to 15-minute intervals throughout the day.

3. Know your target heart rate. Most healthy individuals can exercise at between 60- 80% of their maxium heart rate. Find the zone where you are going to see the most benefit with the least amount of risk. The chart on Page 45 [Need X-ref] will help measure your resting heart rate.

4. Warm up for 5- 10 minutes by walking at a slow pace and gradually increasing speed until you reach your target heart rate. At the end of

your session, walk slowly for 5- 10 minutes until your heart rate nears pre-exercise levels.

5. Stop walking if you experience pain, dizziness, severe shortness of breath, or any unusual signs or symptoms. If the condition persists, seek medical attention.

6. Drink water before, during, and after your walk. Take a bottle or container of water to avoid dehydration.

7. Add variety by alternating intervals of slow, moderate, and fast paces. You can also walk up hills, on trails, or increase the distance to continue progressing. Never walk while carrying wrist or ankle weights as they can cause unnecessary stress on your joints.

8. Prepare for your environment. That may mean dressing in layers that you can take off as you get warmer, or wearing synthetic fabrics to draw moisture from your skin. Always wear a hat and sunscreen.

9. Choose properly fitted footwear that is supportive and cushioned.

10. Be safe. Walk in a secure area or with a buddy. Carry a cell phone. If you wear a headset, keep the volume low so you can be aware of your surroundings.

Measuring Your Target Heart Rate

How to take your pulse: Place your index and middle finger around the back side of your wrist (approximately one inch down from the top of your wrist on the thumb side). Find your pulse and count for six seconds. Multiply this number by 10. Try to keep this number in your target zone.

Age in Years	Average Maximum Heart Rate	Target Heart Rate for Exercise at 60-80% of Maximum Heart Rate
20	200	120-160
30	190	114-152
40	180	108-144
50	170	102-136
60	160	96-128
70	150	90-120

Stretching, Aerobics, and Strength Training
Keeping It Balanced

A balanced fitness program consists of three components: stretching, aerobics and strength training.

Stretching

Regular stretching can help reduce pain, improve muscle imbalances, and decrease your chance of injury.

Stretching Tips

1. Stretch after exercise, when your muscles are warm and more receptive to deeper stretching.

2. Focus on the muscle you are stretching and keep all the other muscles relaxed.

3. Move into each stretch slowly, until you feel mild tension in the muscle. Never bounce.

4. If you feel pain, you've stretched too far.

5. Breathe deeply, slowly and rhythmically while holding the stretch. Never hold your breath.

6. Hold each stretch for at least 10-30 seconds, then release.

7. A stretch can be repeated several times before moving on to another stretch.

8. After you have held a stretch, relax that muscle group and try to stretch again, going a little further each time.

9. Ideally, you should spend at least 30 minutes three times a week, on flexibility training.

10. The practice of yoga or Pilates will also help enhance flexibility.

Aerobics

Aerobic exercise not only helps you burn calories and lose weight more quickly, but research also shows that those who maintain a long-term aerobic program are more likely to keep the weight off. There are several cardiovascular (aerobic) exercises to choose from and include jogging, brisk walking, swimming, biking, skiing and aerobic dancing, among others.

All aerobic exercise increases your heart rate and breathing. It makes no difference what form of exercise you choose as long as you get your heart rate up. So the best exercise for you is the exercise that you enjoy and do on a regular basis.

Strength Training

Strength training can transform your body into a desirable shape and help defy the aging process. It does not need to be time-consuming or expensive to produce health and fitness benefits. The goal is to develop and maintain a significant amount of muscle mass to increase metabolism.

Strength Training Tips

1. Strength training should be performed 2-3 times a week on alternating days.

2. Perform at least one exercise for each major muscle group each session.

3. Always work from the largest to the smallest muscles when designing your routine.

4. Always warm up with 5-10 minutes of cardiovascular activity—such as walking—prior to strength training.

5. Choose a resistance that you can complete in 8-12 repetitions. If you can't complete eight, the weight or resistance is too heavy. If you can go beyond 12, increase the resistance by 5%.

6. All movements should be controlled. When in doubt, slower is always better. Never sacrifice your form to lift more weight.

7. Rest for approximately 30 seconds between exercises.

8. Use a combination of fitness bands, free weights, machines, or fitness balls.

9. Make your program more challenging by adding more resistance, slowing down the range of motion, changing your exercises, trying new equipment or positions, or varying the angles.

10. One set when performed intensely and with good form is enough to produce results and maximize your time investment.

Physical Activity and Calories Burned

Medical and fitness experts measure physical exertion as a MET value (Metabolic equivalent). This is a multiple of oxygen consumption during rest. 1 MET equals 3.5ml/kg/min., which is the amount of oxygen that a person needs while at rest. For example, 13 METs as a result of an exercise test means the person can exceed his resting oxygen consumption 13 times.

To determine the calories you are expending per hour, multiply your weight in kilograms by the MET value given in the chart below. To find your body weight in kilograms, divide your weight in pounds by 2.2. For example, 150 pounds divided by 2.2 equals 68 kilograms. Multiply this figure by the MET value to determine how many calories you will burn per hour while engaged in that activity. A 150-pound person engaged in an hour of high-impact aerobics would expend 477 calories

MET Value	Physical Activity
6.0	Aerobic Dance, general
7.0	Aerobic Dance, high-impact
5.0	Aerobic Dance, low-impact
7.0	Backpacking
5.5	Ballroom Dancing, fast
3.0	Ballroom Dancing, slow
8.0	Basketball game
4.0	Bicycling > 10 miles per hour, leisure ride

MET Value	Physical Activity
6.0	Bicycling 10-12 miles per hour, slow
8.0	Bicycling 12-14 miles per hour, moderate
10.0	Bicycling 14-16 miles per hour, vigorous
12.0	Bicycling 16-19 miles per hour, racing
16.0	Bicycling > 20 miles per hour, racing
5.0	Bicycling Stationary, light effort
7.0	Bicycling Stationary, moderate effort
12.5	Bicycling Stationary, very vigorous effort
10.5	Bicycling Stationary, vigorous effort
3.0	Bowling
8.0	Calisthenics, heavy effort
4.5	Calisthenics, light or moderate effort, (e.g., push-ups, pull-ups, sit-ups)
8.0	Circuit Training, general
6.0	Elliptical Training, general
5.5	Golf, carrying clubs
4.5	Golf, general
6.5	Horseback Riding, trotting
3.5	House Cleaning, general
7.0	Jogging, general
10.0	Jumping Rope, moderate
10.0	Karate, Kickboxing, Tae Kwan Do, Judo
8.5	Mountain Biking
5.5	Mowing Lawn, general, push mower
7.0	Racquetball, casual
8.0	Rock or Mountain Climbing
7.0	Roller Skating
9.5	Rowing Stationary, general
3.5	Rowing Stationary, light effort
7.0	Rowing Stationary, moderate effort
12.0	Rowing Stationary, very vigorous effort
8.5	Rowing Stationary, vigorous effort
8.0	Running > 5 miles per hour
10.0	Running > 6 miles per hour

MET Value	Physical Activity
11.5	Running > 7 miles per hour
13.5	Running > 8 miles per hour
15.0	Running > 9 miles per hour
9.5	Ski Machine, general
7.0	Skiing, general
8.0	Stair Climbing, general
8.0	Swimming Laps, moderate effort
4.0	Tai Chi
7.0	Tennis, general
3.0	Volleyball, general
3.0	Walking > 3 miles per hour
4.0	Walking > 3.5 miles per hour
4.0	Water Aerobics
6.0	Weight Lifting, machine or free weight, vigorous
4.0	Yoga, Hatha

Chapter Five
THE POCKET DIET MEAL PLAN

How Many Calories Do You Need?

Achieving your ideal weight begins with finding the right balance of exercise and caloric intake. Each person's balance is unique. The best way to find out your personal caloric needs is to have your metabolism tested. Metabolism testing measures the amount of oxygen burned while resting. Testing also calculates how many calories you would burn in a day if you rested the entire day. This test can help you determine how many calories you should be eating each day to maintain, gain or lose weight. To have your metabolism tested locally visit www.healthetech.com/dlrlocator.

You can choose from three meal plans on the Pocket Diet. These depend on your size, *activity level and personal goals.* Meal plans are designed to provide you with the appropriate amounts of carbohydrates, protein, and fat to achieve a weight loss of 1-2 pounds per week.

The Pocket Diet allows you to eat a variety of healthy, tasty foods. However, you must pay close attention to both portion sizes and amount of food you eat.

Meals and the Pocket Diet

The most frequently asked question about the Pocket Diet is: "Do I really have to eat all my meals in a Kangaroo Pocket?"

It's not necessary all the time, but if you want a simple and effective way to control portions while developing healthy eating habits, the pocket bread is the key. This is what the study group discovered. It is also a critical and convenient source of complex carbohydrates and perfect for breakfast, lunch and some dinner meals.

Portion control is the essence of any successful diet, including the Pocket Diet. You can't overfill a pocket like a sandwich or your plate. We believe that you will find, as did the 38 members in the Community Memorial Hospital study, that the Kangaroo pocket is a convenient, healthy and delicious way to eat your favorite foods and control your portions.

However, for meals without bread, or when you want a change, just select another complex carb equivalent to the pocket bread from the "Pocket Bread Equivalent Chart" in the appendix section on page 123.

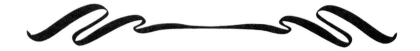

About the Kangaroo Pocket

Kangaroo Pocket bread is a fat-free, wholesome bread made with unbleached white, whole wheat, or whole grain flour. It has a delicious light, hearth-baked flavor that compliments the taste of all foods. The exact nutritional content varies by variety, but a 1.3-ounce whole wheat pocket contains approximately 80 calories and 16 grams of carbohydrates, with 4 grams of fiber, and 3 grams of protein. By comparison, two slices of traditional sandwich bread, bagels, buns or muffins have significantly more calories and carbs than a Kangaroo Pocket.

Substituting a Kangaroo Pocket for traditional sliced bread, bagels or buns can lead to a significant reduction in calories every week.

Basic Meal Plans

The following sample meal plans on page 54 are based on the average number of calories in the pita pocket recipes. Plan-A has 1400 calories; Plan-B, 1800 calories; and Plan-C, 2200 calories.

To determine the meal plan that best fits your body type and activity level, use the following guidelines with a calorie range for the body types described on next page. To obtain your exact caloric requirement and select the appropriate Pocket Diet meal plan, you may want to consult a registered dietitian or visit: www.healthetech.com/dlrlocator.

Increasing physical activity is a key factor in the success of the Pocket Diet. When you first begin the Pocket Diet, you might want to select the pockets that are below the average calorie recipe. As you boost your physical activity, you can incorporate some the higher calorie recipes within the same plan.

Select Meal Plan A (1,200 to 1,600 calories a day) if you are:
- a small woman who exercises regularly
- a small or medium woman who wants to lose weight
- a medium woman who does not exercise much

Select Meal Plan B (1,600 to 2,000 calories a day) if you are:
- a medium woman who exercises regularly
- a large woman who wants to lose weight
- a small man at a healthy weight
- a medium man who does not exercise much
- a medium to large man who wants to lose weight

Select Meal Plan C (2,000 to 2,400 calories a day) if you are:
- a medium to large man who exercises regularly, or has a physically active job
- a large man at a healthy weight
- a large woman who exercises regularly, or has a physically active job

	Plan A 1200 - 1600	Plan B 1600 - 2000	Plan C 2000-2400
A small woman who exercises regularly	■		
A small woman who wants to lose weight	■		
A medium woman who does not exercise much	■		
A medium woman who exercises regularly		■	
A large woman who wants to lose weight		■	
A small man at a healthy weight who exercises regularly		■	
A medium man who does exercise		■	
A medium to large man who wants to lose weight		■	
A medium to large man who exercises regularly, or has a physically active job			■
A large man at a healthy weight			■
A large woman who exercise regularly or has a physically active job			■

Adapted from: National Institute of Health (www.niddk.nih.gov)

Three Meal Plans

Eating a variety of the recipes during the week is important for well-balanced nutrition, and to ensure that not just the higher calorie meals are being consumed.

For beverages, choose water most often. However, 4-8 ounces of 100% fruit juice, skim or lowfat milk, or sugar free soda and tea may be consumed at each meal.

Plan A
Average of 1,400 calories/day

Breakfast	1 Pita Pocket Meal with skim milk	or	1 cup whole grain cereal
Snack			Snack from list
Lunch	1 Pita Pocket Meal	with	1 cup raw veggies
Snack	1 Pita Pocket Meal	or	Snack from list
Dinner	2 Pita Pocket Meals with 1/2 cup veggies	or	3 oz lean protein 3⁄4 cup whole grain starch 1 cup vegetables 2 tsp fat (olive oil, butter or dressing)
Snack			Snack from List

Plan B
Average of 1,800 calories/day

Breakfast	1 Pita Pocket Meal	or	1.5 cup whole grain cereal with skim milk
Snack	1 Pita Pocket Meal	or	Snack from list
Lunch	2 Pita Pocket Meals	with	1 cup raw veggies
Snack	1 Pita Pocket Meal	or	Snack from list
Dinner	2 Pita Pocket Meals	or	5 oz lean protein With 1/2 cup veggies 1 cup whole grain starch 1 cup vegetables 2 tsp fat (olive oil, butter or dressing)
Snack			Snack from list

Plan C
Average of 2,200 calories/day

Breakfast	2 Pita Pocket Meals	or	2 cup whole grain cereal with skim milk
Snack	2 Pita Pocket Meals	or	Snack from list
Lunch	2 Pita Pocket Meals	with	1 cup raw veggies
Snack	2 Pita Pocket Meal	or	Snack from list
Dinner	2 Pita Pocket Meals With 1/2 cup veggies	or	6 oz lean protein 1 cup whole grain starch 1 cup vegetables 1 Tbs fat (olive oil, butter or dressing)
Snack			Snack from list

Sample Meal Plan - Food Selections

Meal Plan: Breakfast	A – 1,400	B – 1,800	C – 2,200
Recipe	1-Veggie scramble	1-Date walnut Spread	2-Bacon Cheese Tomato
Pocket Bread	1-Pocket bread	1-Pocket bread	2-Pocket bread
AM Snack	1 small banana	1 orange 1/2 cup low fat cottage cheese	1 grapefruit 1/2 cup low fat cottage cheese
Lunch			
Recipe	1-Chicken salad	2-Tuna salad	2-Shrimp salad
Pocket Bread	1-Pocket bread & baked potato chips	2-Pocket bread	2-Pocket bread
Vegetable	1 cup raw veggies	1 cup raw veggies	1 cup raw veggies
PM Snack	1/4 cup almonds	1/2 cup yogurt 1 apple	1/2 cup mixed nuts and seeds 1 banana
Dinner			
Recipe	2-Philly cheese steak	2-Chicken stir fry	2-Garbanzo chicken
Pocket Bread	2-Pocket bread	2-Pocket bread	2-Pocket bread
Vegetable	1/2 cup veggies	1/2 cup veggies (in stir fry)	1 cup veggies
PM Snack	3 graham crackers	1/4 cup nuts	1/2 cup sherbet

Eat foods in moderation. Not all foods within a category are created equal. For example, whole, fresh apples should be consumed more often than apple pie, and a person should try to get most of their dairy intake from low-fat milk instead of cream cheese or other high-fat dairy products.

Some tips on making selections include:

- Make half your grains whole grains
- Vary your veggies
- Focus on fruit
- Consume calcium rich foods (low fat dairy products, enriched soy products, green leafy vegetables, etc.)
- Go lean with protein (turkey and chicken breasts, egg whites, tofu, fish, etc.).

Still Hungry?

If you are still hungry after meals and between snacks while following your meal plan, increase your vegetables. Vegetables are full of water and high in fiber. Although they fill you up, they are low in calories. Try some of the veggies below:

Cucumbers	Broccoli
Asparagus	Spinach
Kale	Tomato
Celery	Carrots
Peppers	Sugar snap peas
Brussels sprouts	Cauliflower
Cabbage	Lettuce

Managing Snacks

The best way to ensure that you are eating the healthiest snacks is to have them readily available. Following are some tips for healthy snacking:

- Stock your pantry at home and your drawers at work.
- Eat a wide variety of these snacks.
- Eat something every 3-4 hours, and never wait until you are so hungry that you will eat anything.
- Also make sure you watch your portions.
- Eat the snacks one hour before your main meals to suppress your appetite.

Best Snack List

Snack Foods	Serving Size Average Calories	Serving Tips & Comments
Fresh Fruits Apple, orange, tangerine, pear, Kiwi, banana, cantaloupe, honey dew, plums, All berries, nectarine, mango, apricots, grapes (17 per serving)	1 med. size fruit /or 1/2 cup = 80 calories	Eat a variety of all these healthy fruits 2-3 per day
Veggies baby carrots, celery sticks, pickles, cauliflower, broccoli, cucumbers kohlrabi, fresh string beans, bell peppers… any fresh, non-starchy veggies you like!	1 cup = 80 calories	These are the most nutritious low calorie snacks you can eat. Dip them in a no fat low calorie dressing if you desire.
Nuts almonds, walnuts, unsalted roasted peanuts, sunflower seeds, toasted soy beans Pop Corn (easy salt no butter)	1/4 cup, or approx. 15 nuts = 75 calorie 3 cups = 90 calories	Tip: Buy these nuts in large 24 oz. bags and mix them all together in equal portions. Add some raisins for a bit of sweetness and fiber.
Dried fruit Apricots, figs, date, raisins	1/4 cup, or 4-5 pieces = 60 calories	These are hi- fiber, but high in natural sugar.
Yogurt Choose no fat low sugar variety	1/2 cup = 80 calories or 110 with a little fruit	Mix in fresh cut fruit: berries, pear, nectarine, peach
Cottage Cheese Choose no fat, or 2% fat	1/2 cup = 80-100 calories	Mix in low sugar fruit cocktail, or fresh cut peaches, nectarine
Frozen yogurt Fat Free, or Regular	1/3 cup = 80 calories	Try 1/4 cup, it maybe just enough to satisfy that sweet tooth after dinner
Sorbet / Sherbet	1/3 cup = 80 calories	

Planning Your Meals

As you familiarize yourself with the meal plans, please keep the following in mind:

1. A serving/portion size for the majority of recipes is approximately 3 ounces by weight, or 1/3 of a cup by volume, which equals the contents that a Kangaroo Pocket can hold. If the portion serving size is less or more than that amount, it will be specified in the nutritional information in a recipe.

2. The recipe calories-per-serving listed in each meal plan are based on the average calories-per-serving for all the recipes in each meal section. Each recipe varies in caloric content. It assumes you are eating a variety of the recipes, which is recommended. We used an average of 85 calories for one Kangaroo Pocket which is not included in the calorie total for the recipe.

3. You can adjust the meal plans to a certain calorie level for your specific body and desired weight loss. The food quantity lists in this chapter should help with this.

4. Drink plenty of water. You can also have limited amounts of nonfat or lowfat (1%) milk and natural fruit juices (100% juice), but be sure and check the serving size, and incorporate the calorie count into your overall daily total. Diet soft drinks, ice tea, hot tea, coffee, or any others that contains no sugar are allowed. Avoid beverages with empty calories such as sweetened tea and colas.

5. Choose healthy snack foods from the "Best Snack List" on page 58.

6. You may substitute other complex carbs for the pocket bread. Check the pocket bread equivalent chart in the appendix on page 123.

7. Focus on eating the correct portions for each meal plan.

8. You do not have to eat all the food for each meal in one sitting. Grazing throughout the day is acceptable. Just keep track of what you eat.

9. Eating all types of foods is important for well-balanced nutrition, and for your enjoyment.

Make sure you eat a variety of the recipes during the week. Remember to eat slowly and savor your food. It takes your body 15-20 minutes to feel satisfied after you start eating.

Tips for Pocket Plan Success:

- Plan your weekly meals (very important).
- Stock your pantry with the foods on the plan. Get rid of unhealthy convenience food.
- Prepare enough food so that you will have leftovers for the next day.
- Do not worry if you overeat on any given day, just get back on track the next day. Missing one day will not have a significant impact on your diet.
- Focus on maintaining a daily / weekly average of your calorie goal.
- Stay within the total calories allowed for each week.

The Pocket Diet
Perfect Portion Control that Works!

Recipes

Meal Section Index

Breakfast Recipes	Pages 64-75
Ham & Egg Cheese Pocket	64
Veggie Scramble Pocket	65
Mediterranean Egg Salad	66
Broccoli Quiche Pocket	67
Date & Walnut Spread	68
Crunchy Key Lime Banana Pocket	69
Creamy Summer Berry Pocket	70
Swiss Mushroom & Egg Pocket	71
Lox & Cream Cheese Pocket	72
Bacon Cheese Tomato Pocket	73
Avocado Tomato & Yogurt Pocket	74
Peanut Butter & Banana Pocket	75

Lunch Recipes	Pages 77-94
Tuna Salad Supreme	77
Chicken Sesame Pocket	78
Gourmet Turkey Pocket	79
Gourmet Chicken Salad	80
Apple Walnut Tuna Salad	81
Grecian Salad Pocket	82
Cheesy Fruit Pocket	83
Dill Shrimp Salad	84
Garden Lovers Bean Sauté	85
Crabby Salad Pocket	86
Crunchy Pork Pocket	87
Cheesy Salad Pocket	88
Shrimp Avacado Pocket	89
Black Bean Salad	90
Hummus	91
Tabouleh	92
Reuben Pocket	93
Tomato Basil Pocket	94

Dinner Recipes	Pages 96-117
Chicken Fajita Pocket	96
Beef Fajita Pocket	97
Pork Stir Fry	98
Philly Cheese Steak Pocket	99
Chicken Stir Fry	100
Beef Stir Fry	101
Grilled Salmon & Veggies	102
Grilled Halibut & Veggies	103
Grilled Pork & Root Veggies	104
Pork Tenderloin & Apple Pocket	105
Cabbage & Beef	106
Meat Loaf Lean & Hearty	107
Not So Sloppy Joe Pocket	108
Mediterranean Beef Pocket	109
Garbonzo Chicken Pocket	110
Beef & Mushroom Barley Soup	111
Sandy's Old Country Lentil	112
Sweet Potato & Chick Pea Stew	113
Spinach & Feta Pasta	114
Roasted Vegetables	115
Broccoli and Tofu Pocket	116
Chapatti Pocket	117

Note: *All nutritional information for this recipe does NOT include the Pita Pocket since the quantity consumed varies by recipe and meal plan. A standard one-half 6" pita pocket has approximately 80-90 calories each. Please refer to the food label on the pita packaging to get an accurate count. If you follow the Pocket Diet Meal Plan, you do not have to keep track of your calories as long as you stay within the plan's recommendations.*

Breakfast

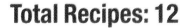

Total Recipes: 12

Lowest Calorie: 82
Highest Calorie: 204

Average: 132

Pocket Bread Calorie: 85

*For all meals, don't forget to eat a variety of the
recipes. This ensures a good nutritional balance and
that you consume the proper caloric average.*

Ham, Egg & Cheese Pocket

Servings: 1   Time: 5 minutes

Ingredients

1/3 cup egg whites
1/4 cup lean ham; diced
2 Tbsp. cheddar or monterey jack cheese; low fat & shredded

1. Coat skillet with nonstick cooking spray & place on medium heat.
2. Warm ham for one minute.
3. Add egg whites & cheese.
3. Stir until firm. Salt & pepper to taste.
4. Fill pocket & serve.

Nutritional Information (per serving)

Calories	115	Cholesterol	20mg	Fiber	0g
Total Fat	3g	Sodium	732mg	Sugar	Trace
Saturated Fat	1g	Carbohydrates	2g	Protein	22g

Note: *For pita pocket bread nutritional information, see page 62*

Helpful Hints

* You may substitute 1 whole egg. This would add 4g of fat, 2 g saturated fat, 36 calories, 270 mg cholesterol, 16 mg sodium, 4 g protein to the nutritional information of any recipe using egg whites.

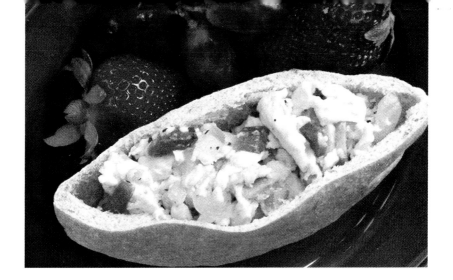

Veggie Scramble Pocket

Servings: 1 Time: 10 minutes

Ingredients

1/3 cup egg whites
1/2 cup mixed bell peppers (red, green & yellow); diced
1/4 medium onion; diced
3 medium mushrooms; diced
2 Tbsp. cheddar or monterey
jack cheese; low fat & shredded

1. Coat skillet with nonstick cooking spray & place on medium heat.
2. Sauté veggies for 3-4 minutes or until tender.
3. Add eggs and cheese; stir until egg whites are firm.
4. Salt & pepper to taste.
5. Fill pocket & serve.

Nutritional Information (per serving)

Calories	106	Cholesterol	3mg	Fiber	2g
Total Fat	2g	Sodium	247mg	Sugar	5g
Saturated Fat	1g	Carbohydrates	7g	Protein	15g

Note: For pita pocket bread nutritional information, see page 62

Helpful Hints

* Reduce prep time each morning by having a supply of refrigerated diced veggies ready to use for a variety of breakfast egg recipes.

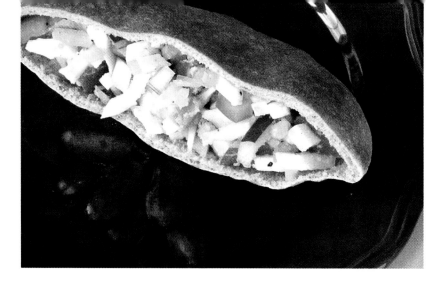

Mediterranean Egg Salad

Servings: 1   Time: 5 minutes

Ingredients

1 hard boiled egg; diced
2 Tbsp. green bell pepper; diced
1 Tbsp. olive oil
1 tsp. onion; diced

1.   Mix egg, veggies and oil in a small bowl.
2.   Salt & pepper to taste.
3.   Fill pocket & serve.

Nutritional Information (per serving)

Calories	203	Cholesterol	212mg	Fiber	1g
Total Fat	19g	Sodium	63mg	Sugar	1g
Saturated Fat	3g	Carbohydrates	2g	Protein	6g

Note: *For pita pocket bread nutritional information, see page 62*

Broccoli Quiche Pocket

Servings: 1   Time: 10 minutes

Ingredients

1/3 cup egg whites
1/3 cup broccoli; chopped
2 Tbsp. cottage cheese; 1% fat
1 Tbsp. onion; minced
1 Tbsp. parmesan cheese; grated

1. Coat skillet with nonstick cooking spray & place on medium heat.
2. Add onions & cook until soft.
3. Mix egg & parmesan cheese in a bowl and cook for 1 minute.
4. Then add broccoli & cottage cheese; stir lightly until eggs are firm.
5. Salt & pepper to taste.
6. Fill pocket & serve.

Nutritional Information (per serving)

Calories	173	Cholesterol	60mg	Fiber	1g
Total Fat	7g	Sodium	550mg	Sugar	3g
Saturated Fat	1g	Carbohydrates	8g	Protein	19g

Note: *For pita pocket bread nutritional information, see page 62*

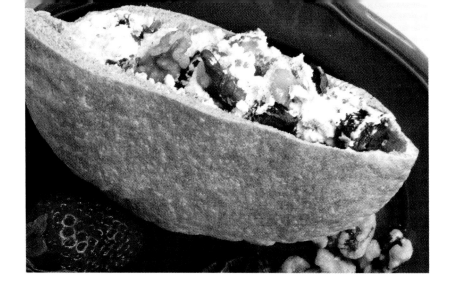

Date & Walnut Spread

Servings: 4   Time: 5 minutes

Ingredients

4 oz. whipped cream cheese; low fat
1/3 cup pitted dates; chopped
1/4 cup walnuts; chopped
1 tsp. cinnamon

1. Mix the dates, walnuts and cream cheese.
2. Sprinkle with cinnamon.
3. Spread 2 tablespoons into pocket and serve.

Nutritional Information (per serving)

Calories	155	Cholesterol	16mg	Fiber	2g
Total Fat	9g	Sodium	84mg	Sugar	9g
Saturated Fat	3g	Carbohydrates	14g	Protein	5g

Note: *For pita pocket bread nutritional information, see page 62*

Helpful Hints

* Double this recipe and keep extra on hand.
  Keeps for 2 weeks in your refrigerator.

Crunchy Key Lime Banana Pocket

Servings: 1 Time: 3 minutes

Ingredients

1/2 banana; sliced
3 Tbsp. key lime pie yogurt; fat free (no sugar added)
1 Tbsp. crunchy wheat & barley cereal or granola

1. Mix yogurt with banana and cereal.
2. Fill pocket & serve.

Nutritional Information (per serving)

Calories	86	Cholesterol	1mg	Fiber	2g
Total Fat	Trace	Sodium	40mg	Sugar	10g
Saturated Fat	Trace	Carbohydrates	1g	Protein	3g

Note: For pita pocket bread nutritional information, see page 62

This makes a delicious
morning or afternoon snack

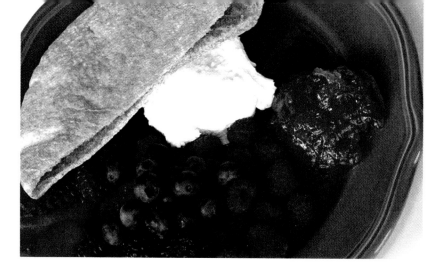

Creamy Summer Berry Pocket

Servings: 1 Time: 3 minutes

Ingredients

1/2 cup fresh berries (raspberry, strawberry, blueberry or blackberry)
1 Tbsp. whipped cream cheese; low fat
1 Tbsp. sugar-free preserves (use a matching berry preserve)

1. Spread inside of pocket with cream cheese.
2. Spread the other inside pocket with the preserve.
3. Add the berries & serve.

Nutritional Information (per serving)

Calories	82	Cholesterol	8mg	Fiber	2g
Total Fat	3g	Sodium	45mg	Sugar	10g
Saturated Fat	1g	Carbohydrates	13g	Protein	2g

This makes a refreshing and healthy desert

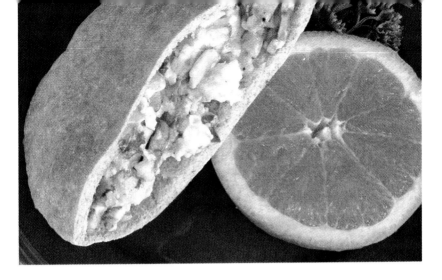

Swiss Mushroom Egg Pocket

Servings: 1 Time: 3 minutes

Ingredients

1/3 cup egg whites
1/3 cup mushrooms, (your choice) chopped
2 Tbsp. swiss cheese; shredded & low fat
1 Tbsp. parsley; chopped (optional)

1. Coat skillet with nonstick cooking spray; place on medium heat.
2. Sauté mushrooms for 3-4 minutes or until tender.
3. Add egg, cheese and parsley; stir until firm.
4. Salt & pepper to taste.
5. Fill pocket & serve.

Nutritional Information (per serving)

Calories	74	Cholesterol	5mg	Fiber	Trace
Total Fat	1g	Sodium	170mg	Sugar	0g
Saturated Fat	Trace	Carbohydrates	2g	Protein	13g

Note: For pita pocket bread nutritional information, see page 62

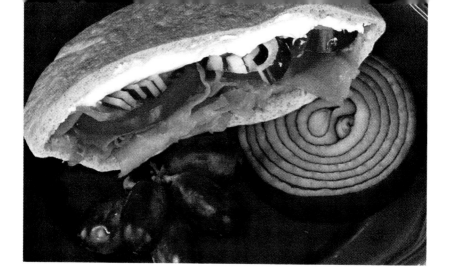

Lox & Cream Cheese Pocket

Servings: 1 Time: 3 minutes

Ingredients

2.5 oz. salmon; unsalted lox
1/2 medium tomato; sliced
1 Tbsp. cream cheese; low fat
1 onion slice (optional)

1. Spread cream cheese in pocket.
2. Add salmon, tomato, onion and serve.

Nutritional Information (per serving)

Calories	141	Cholesterol	24mg	Fiber	1g
Total Fat	6g	Sodium*	—	Sugar	3g
Saturated Fat	2g	Carbohydrates	6g	Protein	15g

* Depends on Salmon variety

Note: *For pita pocket bread nutritional information, see page 62*

Helpful Hints

* Add a touch of horseradish or capers to spice up this recipe.

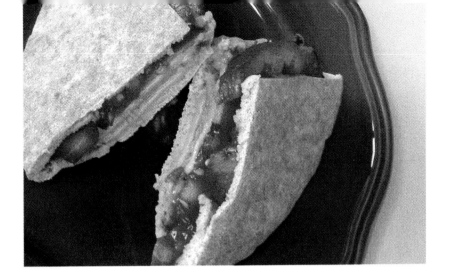

Bacon, Cheese & Tomato Pocket

Servings: 1 Time: 3 minutes

Ingredients

2 oz. cheddar cheese; low fat (monterey jack, provolone, or swiss)
2 oz. canadian bacon or ham
2 tomato slices

1. Heat meat in microwave for 10 seconds on high.
2. Layer cheese, tomato and meat in pocket.
3. Toast the filled pocket on med-high and serve.

Nutritional Information (per serving)

Calories	176	Cholesterol	42mg	Fiber		Trace
Total Fat	7g	Sodium*	500mg	Sugar		2g
Saturated Fat	3g	Carbohydrates	4g	Protein		24g

* Approx. Depends on Meat

Note: *For pita pocket bread nutritional information, see page 62*

Helpful Hints

* Alternate preparation: Sauté bacon in pan for one minute on medium heat (30 sec. each side).

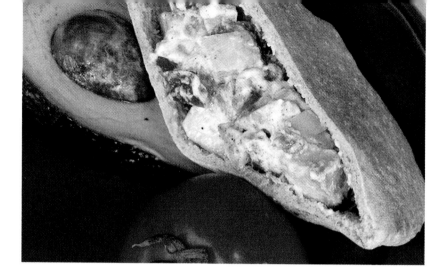

Avocado, Tomato & Yogurt Pocket

Servings: 2 Time: 5 minutes

Ingredients

1 avocado; diced
1 small tomato; diced
2 Tbsp. plain yogurt; low fat
Seasoning salt

1. Mix ingredients in a small bowl.
2. Salt & pepper to taste.
3. Fill pocket & serve.

Nutritional Information (per serving)

Calories	172	Cholesterol	1mg	Fiber	5g
Total Fat	15g	Sodium*	27mg	Sugar	3g
Saturated Fat	2g	Carbohydrates	10g	Protein	3g

Note: For pita pocket bread nutritional information, see page 62

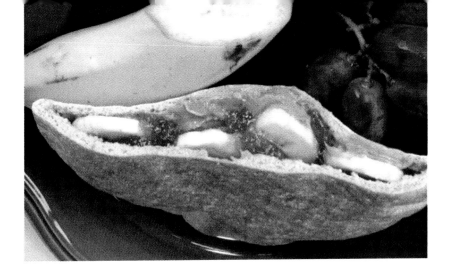

Peanut Butter & Banana Pocket

Servings: 1 Time: 2 minutes

Ingredients

1/2 banana; sliced
1 Tbsp. peanut butter; low fat
1 Tbsp. sugar-free fruit preserve (your choice)

1. Spread peanut butter in pocket.
2. Add preserves, banana and serve.

Nutritional Information (per serving)

Calories	175	Cholesterol	0mg	Fiber	3g
Total Fat	6g	Sodium	95mg	Sugar	17g
Saturated Fat	1g	Carbohydrates	28g	Protein	4g

Note: For pita pocket bread nutritional information, see page 62

This is an ideal afternoon snack and appetite suppressor

Lunch

Total Recipes: 18

Lowest Calorie: 82
Highest Calorie: 204

Average: 132

Pocket Bread Calorie: 85

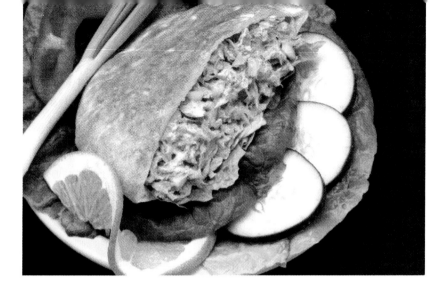

Tuna Salad Supreme

Servings: 4   Time: 15 minutes

Ingredients

6 oz. albacore white tuna in water; drained
1/4 cup celery; diced
1/4 cup pickles; diced (or relish)
1/4 cup apple; diced
1/4 cup onion diced
3 Tbsp. mayonnaise; low fat
1 tsp. horseradish

1. Mix all ingredients in a small bowl.
2. Salt & pepper to taste.
3. Fill pocket & serve.

Nutritional Information (per serving)

Calories	84	Cholesterol	20mg	Fiber	1g
Total Fat	2g	Sodium	398mg	Sugar	2g
Saturated Fat	0g	Carbohydrates	6g	Protein	10g

Note: For pita pocket bread nutritional information, see page 62

Double this recipe, it holds well
for 4-5 days refrigerated

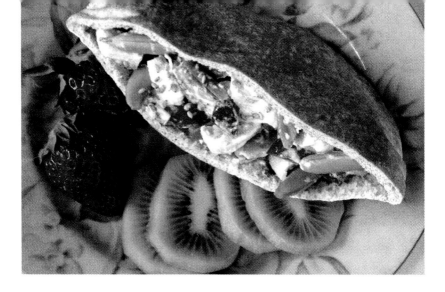

Chicken Sesame Pocket

Servings: 6   Time: 15 minutes

Ingredients

2 skinless-split chicken breasts (10 oz. total); cooked & diced
1/3 cup pea pods or snow peas
1/3 cup red bell pepper; diced
1/4 cup slivered almonds
4 Tbsp. mayonnaise; low fat
2 Tbsp. sesame seeds
2 Tbsp. soy sauce
1/4 Tbsp. ginger; ground

1. Mix mayonnaise, soy sauce, ginger, almonds and sesame seeds to medium bowl; mix well.
2. Stir in chicken, peapods and red pepper.
3. Salt & Pepper to taste.
4. Fill pocket & serve.

Nutritional Information (per serving)

Calories	154	Cholesterol	42mg	Fiber	2g
Total Fat	7g	Sodium	472mg	Sugar	2g
Saturated Fat	1g	Carbohydrates	6g	Protein	17g

Note: For pita pocket bread nutritional information, see page 62

Gourmet Turkey Pocket

Servings: 1   Time: 5 minutes

Ingredients

2 oz. mesquite smoked turkey breast
1 oz. slice of cheese (your choice); low fat
2 slices of tomato
2 lettuce leaves
1 slice of red onion
1 tsp. honey mustard

1.   Fill pocket & serve.

Nutritional Information (per serving)

Calories	179	Cholesterol	45mg	Fiber	1g
Total Fat	6g	Sodium	648mg	Sugar	7g
Saturated Fat	4g	Carbohydrates	9g	Protein	19g

Note: *For pita pocket bread nutritional information, see page 62*

You can substitute your favorite lean deli meats

Gourmet Chicken

Servings: 6 Time: 15 minutes

Ingredients

2 skinless-split chicken breasts (10 oz.); roasted & diced
1/4cup celery; diced
1/4cup grapes; halved
1/4cup apples diced
1/4 cup walnuts; chopped
4 Tbsp. mayonnaise; low fat

1. Mix all ingredients in a small bowl.
2. Salt & pepper to taste.
3. Fill pocket & serve.

Nutritional Information (per serving)

Calories	135	Cholesterol	42mg	Fiber	1g
Total Fat	6g	Sodium	132mg	Sugar	3g
Saturated Fat	1g	Carbohydrates	6g	Protein	15g

Note: For pita pocket bread nutritional information, see page 62

You can substitute your
favorite lean deli meats

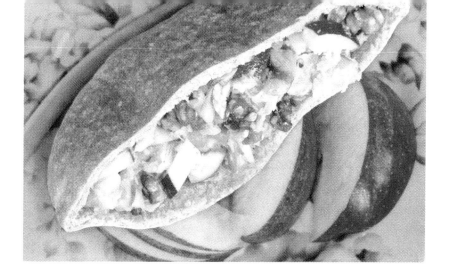

Apple Walnut Tuna

Servings: 4 Time: 15 minutes

Ingredients

6 oz. albacore tuna (in water); drained
1/4 cup celery; diced
1/4 cup walnuts; chopped
1 med. apple; diced
3 Tbsp. mayonnaise; low fat
1 Tbsp. dijon mustard
1 Tbsp. sweet pickle relish

1. Combine all ingredients in a small bowl.
2. Salt & pepper to taste.
3. Fill pocket & serve.

Nutritional Information (per serving)

Calories	150	Cholesterol	20mg	Fiber	2g
Total Fat	7g	Sodium	378mg	Sugar	6g
Saturated Fat	1g	Carbohydrates	11g	Protein	11g

Note: For pita pocket bread nutritional information, see page 62

Try adding dried cranberries to this recipe

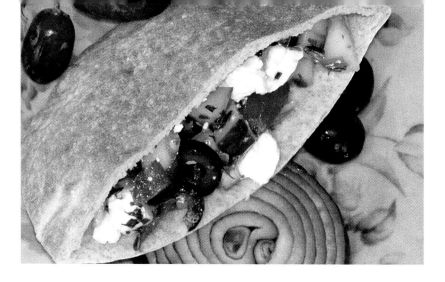

Grecian Salad Pocket

Servings: 8   Time: 15 minutes

Ingredients

4 small cucumbers; peeled & diced
4 small tomato; diced
1 small red onion; diced
1/3 cup crumbled feta cheese
1/4 cup pitted black olives; halved
2 Tbsp. olive oil
1 Tbsp. balsamic vinegar
1 Tbsp. fresh basil; minced
1/2 lemon; freshly squeezed
1/4 tsp. oregano leaves

1. Combine all vegetables in a medium bowl.
2. Mix in oil, vinegar, lemon and seasonings.
3. Salt & pepper to taste.
4. Fill pocket & serve.

Nutritional Information (per serving)

Calories	89	Cholesterol	6mg	Fiber	2g
Total Fat	6g	Sodium	117mg	Sugar	3g
Saturated Fat	2g	Carbohydrates	6g	Protein	3g

Note: For pita pocket bread nutritional information, see page 62

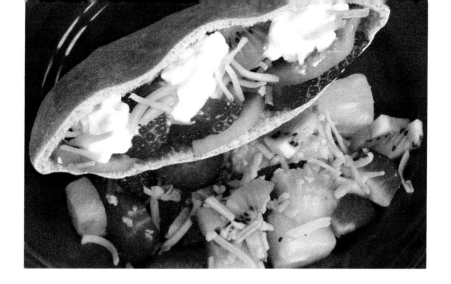

Cheesy Fruit Pocket

Servings: 6   Time: 15 minutes

Ingredients

3 kiwis; peeled and diced
3/4 cup strawberries; sliced
1/4 cup pineapple; diced (if canned, dry thoroughly)
1/2 cup cottage cheese; low fat
4 Tbsp. cheddar cheese; shredded & low fat
1 Tbsp. fresh chives; diced

1. Combine fruit in a bowl.
2. Mix in cottage cheese and cheddar cheese.
3. Fill pocket & serve.

Nutritional Information (per serving)

Calories	102	Cholesterol	6mg	Fiber	2g
Total Fat	2g	Sodium	106mg	Sugar	14g
Saturated Fat	1g	Carbohydrates	16g	Protein	4g

Note: For pita pocket bread nutritional information, see page 62

Another perfect recipe for snack or low calorie refreshing desert

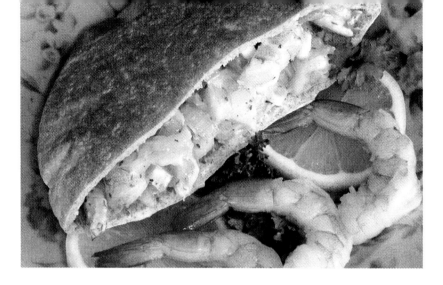

Dill Shrimp

Servings: 10   Time: 15 minutes

Ingredients

2 lbs. cooked shrimp (small or medium size)
3 scallions; chopped
2 celery stalks; chopped
1/4cup plain yogurt; low fat
1/4cup mayonnaise; low fat
1 Tbsp. fresh dill; chopped
2 lemons; juiced
1 lime; juiced

1. Combine all ingredients in large bowl and mix well.
2. Refrigerate until chilled.
3. Fill pocket and serve.

Nutritional Information (per serving)

Calories	76	Cholesterol	2mg	Fiber	2g
Total Fat	1g	Sodium	476mg	Sugar	1g
Saturated Fat	0g	Carbohydrates	5g	Protein	12g

Note: *For pita pocket bread nutritional information, see page 62*

Garden Lovers Bean Sauté

Servings: 12   Time: 25 minutes

Ingredients

12 oz. can black beans; rinse & drain
1 cup fresh bean sprouts; rinse & drain
2 Tbsp. olive oil
1/4 cup green onion; diced
1/4 cup fresh mushrooms; diced
1/4 cup black olives; halved
1/4 cup carrots; shredded
1/4 cup celery; diced
1/4 cup sunflower seeds
1/4 cup fresh chives; diced
1/4 tsp. ground ginger

1. Heat oil in skillet on med-high heat.
2. Sauté bean sprouts, onions, mushrooms and olives;
   until tender (~3 minutes).
3. Reduce heat to low; add carrots, celery, ginger, salt & pepper to taste.
4. Cook for 2-3 minutes.
5. Add black beans and sunflower seeds.
6. Fill pocket with veggies.
7. Top with low fat cheese, sour cream and chives.

Nutritional Information (per serving)

Calories	94	Cholesterol	7mg	Fiber	4g
Total Fat	6g	Sodium	171mg	Sugar	0g
Saturated Fat	2g	Carbohydrates	5g	Protein	4g

Note: *For pita pocket bread nutritional information, see page 62*

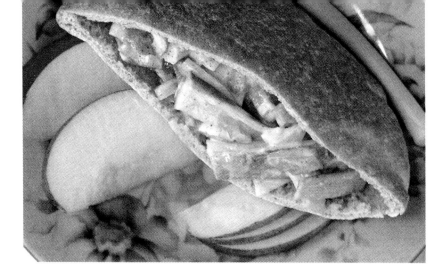

Crabby Salad Pocket

Servings: 6 Time: 15 minutes

Ingredients

12 oz. imitation crab meat; chopped
1/2 cup sour cream; low fat
1/2 cup celery; diced
1/4 cup chutney (store bought);
1/4 cup coconut; flaked
1 tsp. curry powder
1/2 tsp. onion powder
1/2 tsp. ground mustard

1. Mix all ingredients in a small bowl.
2. Salt & pepper to taste.
3. Fill pocket & serve.

Nutritional Information (per serving)

Calories	120	Cholesterol	48mg	Fiber	1g
Total Fat	4g	Sodium	262mg	Sugar	1g
Saturated Fat	3g	Carbohydrates	8g	Protein	13g

Note: *For pita pocket bread nutritional information, see page 62*

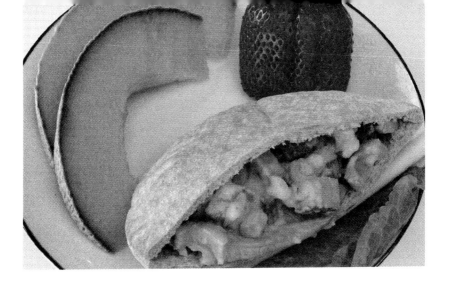

Crunchy Pork Pocket

Servings: 6 Time: 15 minutes

Ingredients

10 oz. (1 1/4 cup) pre-cooked pork; diced
3/4 cup celery; diced
2 Tbsp. mayonnaise; low fat
2 Tbsp. apple sauce
1 scallion; diced

1. Mix all ingredients in a small bowl.
2. Salt & pepper to taste.
3. Fill pocket & serve.

Nutritional Information (per serving)

Calories	129	Cholesterol	40mg	Fiber	0g
Total Fat	8g	Sodium	84mg	Sugar	1g
Saturated Fat	3g	Carbohydrates	3g	Protein	12g

Note: *For pita pocket bread nutritional information, see page 62*

Helpful Hints

* Use leftover pork loin roast or tenderloin.

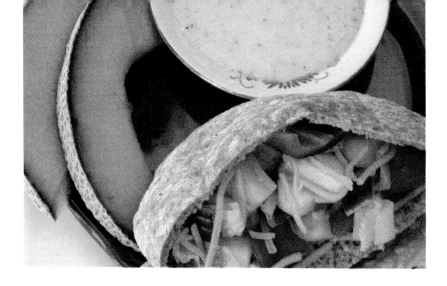

Cheesy Salad Pocket

Servings: 6   Time: 15 minutes

Ingredients

2 small cucumbers; peeled & diced
2 small tomato; diced
1 small red onion; diced
1/2 red bell pepper; diced
1/2 green bell pepper; diced
4 Tbsp. salad dressing (your choice); low fat
3 Tbsp. cheddar cheese; shredded & low fat
1/4 cup alfalfa sprouts (optional)

1.   Combine all ingredients into a bowl.
2.   Salt & pepper to taste.
3.   Fill pocket & serve.

Nutritional Information (per serving)

Calories	56	Cholesterol	0mg	Fiber	2g
Total Fat	1g	Sodium	117mg	Sugar	5g
Saturated Fat	0g	Carbohydrates	10g	Protein	2g

Note: *For pita pocket bread nutritional information, see page 62*

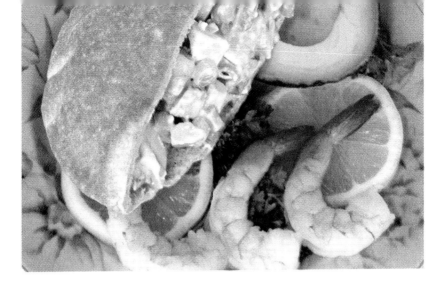

Shrimp & Avocado Pocket

Servings: 8 Time: 15 minutes

Ingredients

1 lb. cooked shrimp; rinse & dry (small or medium size)
2 avocados; diced
3 Tbsp. olive oil
2 medium garlic cloves; minced
2 Tbsp. cilantro; chopped
2 Tbsp. lime juice
1 tsp. ground cumin
1 tsp. jalapeno sauce (optional)

1. Whisk limejuice, garlic, cumin, olive oil, jalapeno sauce and cilantro.
2. Place avocado in mixture; let marinate for 5 minutes.
3. Add cooked shrimp; mix gently.
4. Salt & pepper to taste.
5. Fill pocket and serve.

Nutritional Information (per serving)

Calories	140	Cholesterol	2mg	Fiber	2g
Total Fat	11g	Sodium	278mg	Sugar	0g
Saturated Fat	1g	Carbohydrates	4g	Protein	9g

Note: *For pita pocket bread nutritional information, see page 62*

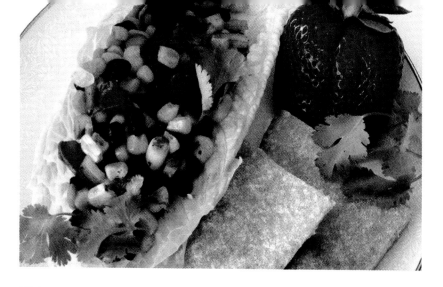

Black Bean Salad

Servings: 8 Time: 15 minutes

Ingredients

12 oz. can black beans; drain & rinse
3 roma tomatoes; diced
2 scallions; diced
1/2 red onion; minced
1/4 cup cilantro leaves; chopped
1/2 cup corn
1 tsp. cumin spice
1 tsp. garlic powder
1 tsp. seasoning salt
1/2 lime; juiced

1. Mix all ingredients into a medium bowl.
2. Squeeze lime over veggies.
3. Stir gently allowing limejuice and spice to coat veggies.
4. Salt & pepper to taste.
5. Fill pocket and serve.

Nutritional Information (per serving)

Calories	66	Cholesterol	0mg	Fiber	4g
Total Fat	1g	Sodium	350mg	Sugar	2g
Saturated Fat	0g	Carbohydrates	12g	Protein	3g

Note: For pita pocket bread nutritional information, see page 62

Hummus (authentic recipe)

Servings: 6 Time: 20 minutes

Ingredients

12 oz. can garbanzo beans (chick peas)
1-2 medium garlic cloves; crushed
2 Tbsp. tahini (ground sesame paste)
1 whole fresh squeezed lemon, or 1/8 cup real lemon juice
1/4 Tbsp. salt

1. Boil garbanzo beans with water from can for 8-10 minutes.
2. Drain 1/3 of the water.
3. Pour beans with water into blender or food processor.
4. Add garlic, tahini, salt and fresh squeezed lemon juice.
5. Puree until you get the smooth consistency of yogurt
   (add water as needed).
6. Place in a shallow bowl or large plate and let cool for 30 minutes.

Nutritional Information (per serving)

Calories	80	Cholesterol	0mg	Fiber	3g
Total Fat	2g	Sodium	462mg	Sugar	3g
Saturated Fat	0g	Carbohydrates	14g	Protein	3g

Note: *For pita pocket bread nutritional information, see page 62*

Helpful Hints

* Authentic Serving Method:
  1. Drizzle 3 Tbsp. of olive oil over top.
  2. Sprinkle with paprika and garnish with cucumber, tomato, pickles, radish and olives. Note: The olive oil adds calories and good fats: approximately 60 calories and 7 grams of fat per serving. Toast the pockets and cut into quarter pieces for dipping. Alternatively, spread hummus into pocket and add veggies or mediterranean beef (see dinner recipe).
* Optional Ingredients:
  Add 1 small jalapeno pepper (remove seeds), and or cilantro.
  Good for 7 days refrigerated.

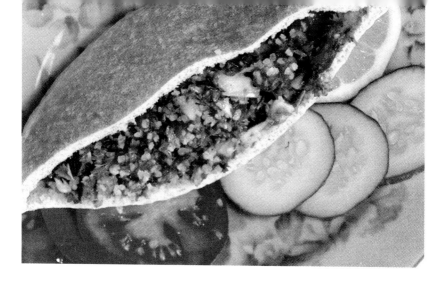

Tabouleh (authentic recipe)

Servings: 8 Time: 30 minutes

Ingredients

3 medium firm tomato; diced (Roma are best)
3 scallions; diced
2 medium cucumbers; peeled & diced
1 large green bell pepper; diced
1 cup parsley; chopped finely
1 cup bulgur-medium (cracked wheat)
1 lemon; freshly squeezed
1/4 cup olive oil

1. Soak bulgar with 1/2 cup of water in a medium bowl.
2. Let it soak for 15 minutes.
3. Drain excess water.
4. Mix lemon juice with olive oil in a separate small bowl.
5. Add lemon juice mixture to bowl with bulgur.
6. Add remaining ingredients; mix well.
7. Salt & pepper to taste.
8. Fill pocket & serve.

Nutritional Information (per serving)

Calories	109	Cholesterol	0mg	Fiber	3g
Total Fat	7g	Sodium	156mg	Sugar	3g
Saturated Fat	1g	Carbohydrates	12g	Protein	3g

Note: *For pita pocket bread nutritional information, see page 62*

Reuben Pocket

Servings: 4 Time: 15 minutes

Ingredients

12 oz. thin sliced corned beef
1 Cup prepared Sauerkraut; warmed in sauce pan
4 Tbsp. Spicy mustard
4 Tbsp. Thousand Island Dressing
4 slices Swiss cheese

1. Spread 1 Tbs. Mustard on bottom and 1 Tbs.
    Thousand Island dressing inside each pocket.
2. Fill pocket with 3 oz. of Corned Beef, add warmed
    Sauerkraut and 1 slice Swiss cheese.
3. Place in large nonstick skillet on low cover and warm
    each side for 1 minute until cheese melts.
4. Fill pockets and serve.

Nutritional Information (per serving)

Calories	253	Cholesterol	53mg	Fiber	2g
Total Fat	15g	Sodium	1906mg	Sugar	3g
Saturated Fat	6g	Carbohydrates	9g	Protein	23g

Note: For pita pocket bread nutritional information, see page 62

Tomato Basil Pocket

Servings: 2 Time: 5 minutes

Ingredients

1 Vine ripened large tomato; sliced
4 Fresh basil leaves; diced
2 Thin slices of red onion
2 Slices of cheese; your choice
A few splash of balsamic vinegar

1. Toast the Pita pocket on low / med.
2. Layer tomato slices sprinkle basil and balsamic vinegar.
3. Add onion and cheese and serve.
4. Fill pockets and serve.

Nutritional Information (per serving)

Calories	105	Cholesterol	20mg	Fiber	1g
Total Fat	7g	Sodium	309mg	Sugar	4g
Saturated Fat	4g	Carbohydrates	6g	Protein	6g

Note: For pita pocket bread nutritional information, see page 62

Dinner

Total Recipes: 22

Lowest Calorie: 82
Highest Calorie: 204

Average: 132

Pocket Bread Calorie: 85

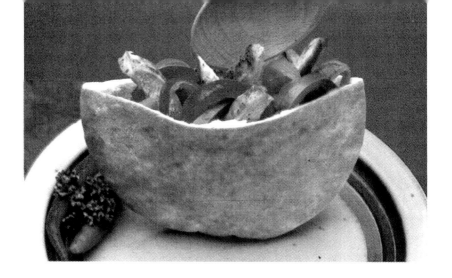

Chicken Fajita Pocket

Servings: 6   Time: 25 minutes

Ingredients

3 skinless-split chicken breasts (12 oz. total)
1 green bell pepper; sliced into long strips
1 medium onion; sliced
1 Tbsp. canola oil
1 tsp. chicken fajita seasoning

1. Heat oil in large skillet on med-high heat for 1 minute.
2. Season whole breast; sauté until brown (3-4 min. each side).
3. Remove chicken from pan; slice into 1/2" x 1" strips.
4. Add peppers and onions to pan; cook until tender.
5. Add chicken back to pan and stir with peppers & onion for 1-2 minutes.
6. Fill pocket & serve.

Nutritional Information (per serving)

Calories	125	Cholesterol	50mg	Fiber	1g
Total Fat	4g	Sodium	152mg	Sugar	1g
Saturated Fat	1g	Carbohydrates	3g	Protein	18g

Note: For pita pocket bread nutritional information, see page 62

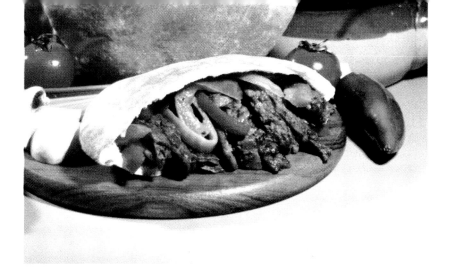

Beef Fajita Pocket

Servings: 6 Time: 25 minutes

Ingredients

12 oz. lean sirloin or beef tenderloin
1 green bell pepper; sliced into 1"strips
1 medium onion sliced
2 Tbsp. canola oil
1 tsp. beef fajita seasoning

1. Heat oil in large skillet on med-high heat for 1 minute.
2. Season beef and sauté until browned (2-3 minute each side).
3. Remove beef from pan; slice into thin 1" strips.
4. Add peppers and onions to pan; cook until tender.
5. Add beef back to pan; stir with peppers and onion for 1-2 minutes.
6. Fill pocket & serve.

Nutritional Information (per serving)

Calories	214	Cholesterol	40mg	Fiber	1g
Total Fat	18g	Sodium	152mg	Sugar	1g
Saturated Fat	6g	Carbohydrates	3g	Protein	10g

Note: *For pita pocket bread nutritional information, see page 62*

Pork Stir Fry

Servings: 6 Time: 25 minutes

Ingredients

12 oz. pork tenderloin; cut into 1/2" pieces
1 red bell pepper; cut into 1"strips
1 yellow bell pepper
1 cup mushroom (your choice); sliced
1 cup bean sprouts
2 small garlic cloves; crushed
1/2 cup onion; chopped
1 Tbsp. canola oil
1/4 cup of your favorite pork stir fry marinade (reduced sodium)

1. Place pork strips into a small bowl with marinade for at least 10 minutes*.
2. Heat oil in large fry pan on med-high heat for 1 minute.
3. Add pork and garlic; stir constantly for 4-6 minutes.
4. Add remaining vegetables.
5. Stir for 8-10 minutes or until veggies become tender.
6. Add soy sauce to taste.
7. Fill pocket & serve.

*The longer the meat sits in the marinade, the more flavor it will absorb.

Nutritional Information (per serving)

Calories	134	Cholesterol	37mg	Fiber	1g
Total Fat	5g	Sodium	550mg	Sugar	4g
Saturated Fat	1g	Carbohydrates	9g	Protein	13g

Note: For pita pocket bread nutritional information, see page 62

Helpful Hint

* Use frozen vegetable mix if you are time-crushed.

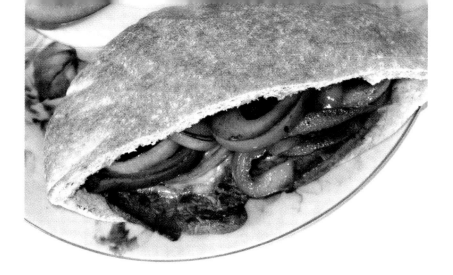

Philly Cheese Steak Pocket

Servings: 1 Time: 15 minutes

Ingredients

2 oz. beef tenderloin; 2 pieces sliced 1/2" thin
1/2 green bell pepper; sliced into long strips
1/2 small onion; sliced
1 oz. provolone cheese; low fat
1 Tbsp. olive oil

1. Heat oil in skillet on med-high heat for 1 minute.
2. Add meat; cook each side for 1 minute.
3. Remove meat from pan on to a plate; top with cheese.
4. Cover plate with lid of pan or another plate to keep meat warm.
5. Add veggies to same pan; stir until tender.
6. Salt & pepper to taste.
7. Fill pocket & serve.

Nutritional Information (per serving)

Calories	313	Cholesterol	56mg	Fiber	3g
Total Fat	22g	Sodium	151mg	Sugar	4g
Saturated Fat	9g	Carbohydrates	12g	Protein	21g

Note: For pita pocket bread nutritional information, see page 62

Chicken Stir Fry

Servings: 6   Time: 25 minutes

Ingredients

3 skinless-split chicken breasts (12 oz. total); cut into small strips 1/2" pieces
1 red bell pepper; cut into
1" strips
1 yellow bell pepper
1 cup mushroom (your choice); sliced
1 cup 8 oz. bean sprouts
2 small garlic cloves; crushed
1/2 cup onion; cut into strips
1 Tbsp. canola oil
1/4 cup of your favorite chicken stir fry marinade (low sodium)

1. Place chicken strips into a small bowl with marinade for at least 10 minutes*.
2. Heat oil in large fry pan on medium heat for 1 minute.
3. Add chicken and garlic; stir constantly for 5-7 minutes.
4. Add remaining vegetables.
5. Stir constantly for 8-10 minutes or until veggies become tender.
6. Add soy sauce & pepper to taste.
7. Fill pocket & serve.

*The longer the meat sits in the marinade, the moreflavor it will absorb.

Nutritional Information (per serving)

Calories	173	Cholesterol	48mg	Fiber	1g
Total Fat	7g	Sodium	550mg	Sugar	3g
Saturated Fat	1g	Carbohydrates	8g	Protein	19g

Note: For pita pocket bread nutritional information, see page 62

Helpful Hints

* To clean chicken: remove from package and rinse chicken thoroughly with cold water. Dry chicken with paper towel.

* Time-Saving Tip: Use frozen vegetable mix if you are time-crushed.

Beef Stir Fry

Servings: 6 Time: 25 minutes

Ingredients

12 oz. beef tenderloin or sirloin steak; cut into 1/2" pieces
1 red bell pepper; cut into 1" strips
1 yellow bell pepper
1 cup mushroom (your choice); sliced
1 cup bean sprouts
2 small garlic cloves; crushed
1/2 cup onion; chopped
1 Tbsp. canola oil
1/4 cup of your favorite beef stir fry marinade (low sodium)

1. Place beef strips into a small bowl with marinade for at least 10 minutes*.
2. Heat oil in large fry pan on medium heat for 1 minute.
3. Add beef and garlic; stir constantly for 3-4 minutes.
4. Add remaining vegetables.
5. Stir constantly for 8-10 minutes or until veggies become tender.
6. Add soy sauce to taste.
7. Fill pocket & serve.

*The longer the meat sits in the marinade, the moreflavor it will absorb.

Nutritional Information (per serving)

Calories	203	Cholesterol	40mg	Fiber	1g
Total Fat	15g	Sodium	550mg	Sugar	1g
Saturated Fat	5g	Carbohydrates	7g	Protein	12g

Note: For pita pocket bread nutritional information, see page 62

Helpful Hint

* Use frozen vegetable mix if you are time-crushed.

Grilled Salmon & Veggies

Servings: 2 Time: 40 minutes

Ingredients

2 salmon filets (4 oz.); skinless (ask your butcher to remove skin)
1 red bell pepper; slice 2" strips
1 yellow bell pepper; slice 2" strips
1 medium onion; quartered
1 cup mushrooms (your choice); halved
1 cup broccoli; sliced to 1" pieces
1 cup cauliflower; sliced to 1" pcs
1 cup of baby carrots
1 fresh lemon
4 Tbsp. olive oil (for veggies)
2 Tbsp. balsamic vinegar/oil dressing
1 Tbsp salt (for cleaning salmon)
Seasoning salt (optional)
Paprika

1. Cover barbeque grate with aluminum foil; preheat to medium.
2. Add all veggies to a large bowl.
3. Season with olive oil, seasoning salt & pepper.
4. Place veggies on foil for 12-15 minutes, stirring occasionally.
5. Remove when semi-tender; place in bowl and cover.

While veggies cook:

1. Soak salmon in small water bowl with 1 Tbsp. of salt water for 10 minutes.
2. Rinse thoroughly; place on paper towel to remove moisture.

After veggies are cooked:

1. Lightly coat same piece of aluminum foil with balsamic vinegar/oil dressing.
2. Season filets lightly with fresh lemon, paprika, salt, pepper.
3. Place filets on foil; cover & cook for 10-12 minutes. Do not turn filet over. Salmon should be slightly pink on inside.

Note: The amount of veggies in this recipe yields 6 servings. Great for leftovers. Serve with a side of wild rice, or pasta (carb side is not included in nutritional nformation)

Nutritional Information (per serving)

Calories	320	Cholesterol	66mg	Fiber	3g
Total Fat	17g	Sodium	383mg	Sugar	5g
Saturated Fat	0g	Carbohydrates	12g	Protein	30g

Note: For pita pocket bread nutritional information, see page 62

Grilled Halibut & Veggies

Substitute with: Tuna, Sword fish, Sea bass, or Shrimp
Servings: 2 Time: 40 minutes

Ingredients

2 halibut filets 4oz.; skinless (ask butcher to remove skin)
1 red bell pepper; slice 2" strips
1 yellow bell pepper
1 medium onion; quartered
1 cup mushrooms (your choice); halved
1 cup broccoli; sliced to 1" pieces
1 cup cauliflower; sliced to 1" pcs
1 cup of baby carrots
1 fresh lemon
4 Tbsp. olive oil
2 Tbsp. balsamic vinegar/oil dressing
1 Tbsp salt
Seasoning salt
Paprika

1. Cover barbeque grate with aluminum foil; preheat to medium.
2. Add veggies to a large bowl.
3. Season with olive oil, seasoning salt & pepper.
4. Place veggies on foil for 12-15 minutes, stirring occasionally.
5. Remove when semi-tender; place in bowl and cover.

While veggies cook:
1. Soak halibut in small bowl of salt water for 10 minutes.
2. Rinse thoroughly; place on paper towel to remove moisture.

After veggies are cooked:
1. Lightly coat same piece of aluminum foil with balsamic vinegar/oil dressing.
2. Season filets with freshly squeezed lemon, paprika, salt, pepper and paprika.
3. Place filets on foil, cover & cook for 10-12 minutes. Do not turn filet over.

Note: The amount of veggies in this recipe yields 6 servings. Great for leftovers. Serve with a side of wild rice, or pasta (carb side is not included in nutritional nformation)

Nutritional Information (per serving)

Calories	320	Cholesterol	13mg	Fiber	3g
Total Fat	6g	Sodium	5mg	Sugar	5g
Saturated Fat	27g	Carbohydrates	12g	Protein	24g

Note: *For pita pocket bread nutritional information, see page 62*

Grilled Pork & Root Veggies

Servings: 4 Time: 40 minutes

Ingredients

1 pork tenderloin, 16 oz.
1/2 cup beets; 1/2" cubes
1/2 cup baby carrots
1/2 cup parsnips; 1/2" cubes
1/2 cup celery; chopped 1/2"
1/2 cup sweet potato; 1/2" cubes
1/2 medium onion; chopped
2 Tbsp. brown sugar
1 Tbsp. olive oil
2 Tbsp. butter

Marinade:
2 garlic cloves; crushed
3 Tbsp. Olive oil
A touch of rosemary
1/2 cup of white wine
1/2 tsp salt, 1/2 tsp pepper

1. Mix ingredients for marinade in a large bowl.
2. Place meat in marinade for 15-20 minutes.
3. Heat oil anf butter in large skillet on medium heat.
4. Add all veggies and brown sugar; stir for 15 minutes until semi soft.
5. Preheat grill to medium.
6. Grill each side of pork for 10-12 minutes.
7. Slice 1/4" thin & serve with veggies.

Nutritional Information (per serving)

Calories	403	Cholesterol	79mg	Fiber	3g
Total Fat	26g	Sodium	150mg	Sugar	9g
Saturated Fat	8g	Carbohydrates	17g	Protein	26g

Note: *For pita pocket bread nutritional information, see page 62*

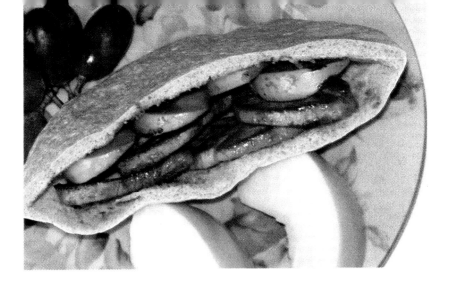

Pork Tenderloin & Apple Pocket

Servings: 2 Time: 15 minutes

Ingredients

6 oz. pork tenderloin; 4 pieces sliced 1/4" thin
3/4 cup apple; peeled and sliced 1/4"
1 Tbsp. apple jelly
1 Tbsp. canola oil
1/2 Tbsp. brown sugar

1. Heat oil in large skillet on med-high heat.
2. Cook pork for 3-4 minutes on each side; salt & pepper to taste.
3. Remove meat; turn heat to medium.
4. Add jelly and brown sugar to skillet; stir well.
5. Add apple and cook on medium heat for 2 minutes.
6. Fill pocket with 2 pieces of pork with apple jelly & serve.

Nutritional Information (per serving)

Calories	233	Cholesterol	56mg	Fiber	1g
Total Fat	12g	Sodium	46mg	Sugar	14g
Saturated Fat	2g	Carbohydrates	15g	Protein	9g

Note: For pita pocket bread nutritional information, see page 62

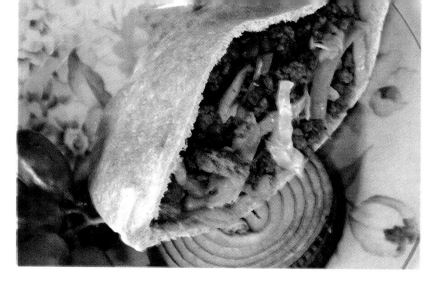

Cabbage & Beef

Servings: 6 Time: 25 minutes

Ingredients

12 oz. ground sirloin (90% lean)
1 cup white cabbage; shredded
1/2 cup onion; diced
2 medium garlic cloves; crushed
2 Tbsp. canola oil

1. Heat oil in large skillet on medium heat.
2. Brown onion and garlic for 3 minutes.
3. Add meat and brown for 3-4 minutes.
4. Turn heat to low; add cabbage.
5. Stir and simmer for 15 minutes.
6. Salt & pepper to taste.
7. Fill pocket & serve.

Nutritional Information (per serving)

Calories	172	Cholesterol	32mg	Fiber	2g
Total Fat	13g	Sodium	60mg	Sugar	0g
Saturated Fat	4g	Carbohydrates	2g	Protein	1g

Note: *For pita pocket bread nutritional information, see page 62*

Meatloaf Lean & Hearty

Servings: 10   Time: 1 hour

Ingredients

2 lbs. ground round (95% lean)
3 egg whites
3/4 cup bread crumbs (plain)
3/4 cup mozzarella cheese; shredded low fat
1/2 cup parsley; chopped
1/4 cup ketchup
1 large onion; chopped fine
1 red bell pepper; diced
1 large tomato; diced
1/2 tsp. pepper
1 tsp. salt

1. Mix all ingredients together in a large bowl.
2. Knead meat gently making sure all ingredients are mixed evenly.
3. Lightly coat 10" bread pan with vegetable oil.
4. Form the meat into pan.
5. Preheat oven to 375°F; bake for one hour.
6. Slice meatloaf 1/2" thin.
7. Place 2 slices in a pocket and serve with roasted veggies.

Nutritional Information (per serving)

Calories	288	Cholesterol	67mg	Fiber	1g
Total Fat	17g	Sodium	500mg	Sugar	2g
Saturated Fat	7g	Carbohydrates	10g	Protein	22g

Note: *For pita pocket bread nutritional information, see page 62*

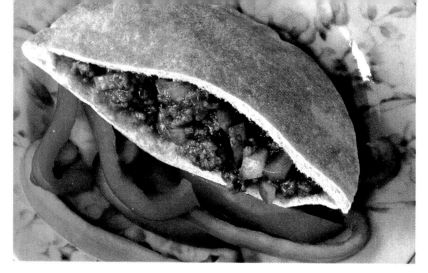

Not So Sloppy Joe Pocket

Servings: 1 Time: 5 minutes

Ingredients

12 oz. ground sirloin (90% lean)
1/2 cup green pepper; diced
1/2 cup onion; diced
1/2 cup celery; diced
1 Tbsp. canola oil
1 cup of sloppy joe sauce (your choice)

1. Heat oil in large skillet on medium heat.
2. Add veggies and sauté for 2 minutes.
3. Add meat and brown meat for 5 minutes.
4. Add sauce; turn heat to low and simmer for 10 minutes.
5. Fill pocket & serve.

Nutritional Information (per serving)

Calories	199	Cholesterol	32mg	Fiber	1g
Total Fat	11g	Sodium	500mg	Sugar	9g
Saturated Fat	4g	Carbohydrates	13g	Protein	12g

Note: *For pita pocket bread nutritional information, see page 62*

www.pocketdiet.com

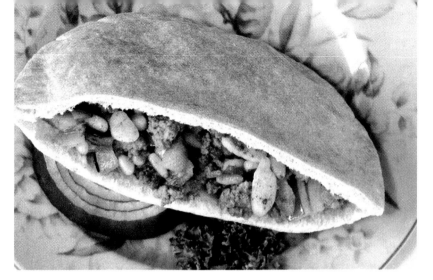

Mediterranean Beef Pocket

Servings: 6 Time: 25 minutes

Ingredients

12 oz. ground sirloin (90% lean)
1 large garlic clove; crushed
1 Tbsp. allspice*
1/4 cup of water

1 medium onion; diced
1/2 cup pine nuts
1 Tbsp. olive oil

*You can substitute a variety of spices to change the flavor: Taco, Cajun, chili etc.

1. Heat oil in large skillet on medium heat.
2. Sauté onion, garlic, and pine nuts for 2-3 minutes.
3. Add meat and spices; brown for 3-4 minutes.
4. Turn heat to low; simmer for 15 minutes, stirring occasionally.
5. Salt & pepper to taste.
6. Fill pocket & serve.

Nutritional Information (per serving)

Calories	226	Cholesterol	32mg	Fiber	1g
Total Fat	17g	Sodium	52mg	Sugar	0g
Saturated Fat	5g	Carbohydrates	5g	Protein	14g

Note: For pita pocket bread nutritional information, see page 62

Helpful Hint

* Spread 2 Tbsp. of hummus in pocket with 2 Tbsp. beef and enjoy!

Garbanzo Chicken Pocket

Servings: 6   Time: 20 minutes

Ingredients

2 chicken breasts skinless-split (10 oz. total); diced
12 oz. can of garbanzo beans (chick peas); rinse & drain
3 scallions; chopped
1 red bell pepper; diced
4 Tbsp. olive oil
1/4 cup parsley; chopped
1/4 cup lemon juice
1 Tbsp. ground cumin
1 tsp. chili powder

1. Season diced chicken breasts with cumin and chili powder.
2. Heat 1 Tbsp. of olive oil in large skillet on med-high heat.
3. Cook chicken for 3-4 minutes on high heat; remove chicken from pan.
4. Add remaining ingredients to pan.
5. Sauté for 3-4 minutes on medium heat.
6. Add chicken back to pan, stir all ingredients for 2-3 minutes.
7. Fill pockets and serve.

Nutritional Information (per serving)

Calories	251	Cholesterol	27mg	Fiber	6g
Total Fat	11g	Sodium	56mg	Sugar	5g
Saturated Fat	1g	Carbohydrates	20g	Protein	17g

Note: For pita pocket bread nutritional information, see page 62

Helpful Hint

* Top with 1 Tbsp. of plain nonfat yogurt and chopped cilantro

Sandy's Beef and Mushroom Barley Soup

Servings: 16 Time: 45 minutes

Ingredients

10 cups of water
2 Tbsp olive oil
2 medium onions diced
4 Beef bullion cubes
2 large carrots sliced
1 cup medium Pearled Barley, uncooked & rinsed
2 cups of mushrooms; sliced (your choice)
1 whole bay leaf

2 Lb. beef stew meat (1/2" pieces)
3 Cloves garlic minced
2 med. tomato; diced (pr 1-16 oz. can)
1 9 oz. bag frozen peas
2 celery stalks clicked

1. Heat oil in a large stockpot on high heat.
2. Brown 1lb. beef at a time.
3. Remove and brown the other lb.
4. Combine browned beef in pot.
5. Reduce heat to medium.
6. Add onions and garlic; cook for 3 minutes.
7. Add 10 cups of water and all other ingredients (except peas.)
8. Bring water to a boil then reduce heat to med/low.
9. Salt & Pepper to taste.
10. Simmer for 1 1/2 hours; stir occasionally.
11. Add peas and simmer for another1/2 hour.

Nutritional Information (per serving)

Calories	173	Cholesterol	60mg	Fiber	1g
Total Fat	7g	Sodium	550mg	Sugar	3g
Saturated Fat	1g	Carbohydrates	8g	Protein	19g

Note: *For pita pocket bread nutritional information, see page 62*

Helpful Hints

* Water may be added if soup gets too thick.
* This soup becomes thicker and richer in flavor the longer it simmers, and it's GREAT the next day!

Sandy's Old Country Lentil

Servings: 12 Time: 30 minutes

Ingredients

10 cups of water
2 med. tomato; diced (or 1-16 oz. can diced tomato)
1 lb. dry lentils; rinse and drain (pick out bad lentils)
2 garlic cloves; minced
2 large carrots; sliced
2 large celery stalks; sliced
2 Tbsp. olive oil
1 large onion; diced
1 tsp. ground cumin
2 chicken boullion cubes
2 tsp. salt
1/2 tsp. pepper

1. Heat oil in a large stockpot on medium heat.
2. Add onions, garlic and spices; sauté until tender.
3. Add tomato and simmer for 10 minutes - stir
4. Add water and boullion cubes, and lentils.
5. Cover and bring to a boil.
6. Reduce heat to mcd/low, simmer 2 hours uncovered - stir occasionally.
7. Add carrots, celery & simmer for 45 minutes - stir occasionaly.

Nutritional Information (per serving)

Calories	163	Cholesterol	0mg	Fiber	12g
Total Fat	3g	Sodium	408mg	Sugar	3g
Saturated Fat	0g	Carbohydrates	19g	Protein	11g

Note: For pita pocket bread nutritional information, see page 62

Sweet Potato & Chick Pea Stew

Servings: 6   Time: 20 minutes

Ingredients

1 16 oz. can of Chick Peas
1 can of whole tomatos, chopped
1 1/2 Lb. of sweet potato peeled, cut 3/4" pieces
1 yellow pepper; diced
2 Garlic cloves; minced
1 cup of cilantro; minced
1 large onion; diced
1 1/2 tsp. ground cumin
3/4 tsp. salt
1/4 tsp. pepper

1. Heat oil in large skillet on medium heat.
2. Add onion, bell pepper and garlic; sauté 5 minutes until tender.
3. Add cumin; stir for 1-2 minutes.
4. Add all other ingredients (except cilantro.)
5. Bring to a light boil.
6. Reduce heat and simmer ~ 15 minutes or until potatoes are tender.
7. Add cilantro and stir for 2 minutes.

Nutritional Information (per serving)

Calories	243	Cholesterol	0mg	Fiber	8g
Total Fat	4g	Sodium	582mg	Sugar	11g
Saturated Fat	0g	Carbohydrates	46g	Protein	6g

Note: For pita pocket bread nutritional information, see page 62

Helpful Hints

*   Serve this over rice, or as a side dish with pork loin roast or grilled pork tenderloin.

Spinach & Feta Pasta

Servings: 8 Time: 20 minutes

Ingredients

2 Tbsp. olive oil
10 oz. fresh spinach
8 oz. of wheat pasta
8 oz. of tomato basil Feta cheese
8 med. tomato; diced
3 Garlic cloves, minced

1. Boil pasta; drain and remove from pot.
2. Heat oil in same pot on high heat.
3. Brown garlic for 2 minutes.
4. Add spinach and tomato; sauté for 2 minutes.
5. Add pasta and Feta cheese; stir it up.

Nutritional Information (per serving)

Calories	228	Cholesterol	25mg	Fiber	2g
Total Fat	11g	Sodium	347mg	Sugar	2g
Saturated Fat	5g	Carbohydrates	26g	Protein	9g

Note: For pita pocket bread nutritional information, see page 62

Helpful Hints

* Serve as a side dish with any meat, or make this recipe with chicken as a complete meal.

* Sauté or grill 3 chicken breasts season with salt & pepper. Slice the cooked chicken breasts, add these after step 3 and heat for 1 minutes before adding the pasta.

Roasted Vegetables

Servings: 10 Time: 1 hour

Ingredients

3 bell peppers (red, yellow, green); sliced 1" x 1"
2 large potatoes; 1" cubed
2 cups cauliflower flowerets
1 cup baby carrots
1 large onion; sliced
1 cup of mushrooms; halved (your choice)
2 jalapenos; de-seeded and sliced (adds flavor with light spice)
4 Tbsp. olive oil

1. Place all ingredients into large bowl; stir well.
2. Make sure olive oil coats all veggies.
3. Place veggies on a large baking pan.
4. Roast in oven at 350°F for 35-45 minutes.

Nutritional Information (per serving)

Calories	97	Cholesterol	0mg	Fiber	3g
Total Fat	6g	Sodium	17mg	Sugar	2g
Saturated Fat	1g	Carbohydrates	11g	Protein	2g

Note: *For pita pocket bread nutritional information, see page 62*

Helpful Hint

* A great side dish with any meat or fish.

Broccoli & Tofu Pocket

Servings: 6 Time: 10 minutes

Ingredients

1 Cup firm tofu; diced
1 Cup broccoli florets; diced
1 Tbsp. olive oil
1/4 cup Flour (for dusting tofu)
Seasonings: Seasoning Salt & Pepper
Thousand island dressing; low fat (you may substitute your favorite)

1. Heat oil in skillet on medium heat.
2. Roll tofu in seasoned flour.
3. Add broccoli to hot oil for 3-4 minutes.
4. Add tofu and cook for 3-4 minutes; stir with broccoli until lightly brown.
5. Fill pocket with tofu and dressing.
6. Fill pockets and serve.

Nutritional Information (per serving)

Calories	97	Cholesterol	1mg	Fiber	1g
Total Fat	7g	Sodium	87mg	Sugar	1g
Saturated Fat	1g	Carbohydrates	4g	Protein	6g

Note: For pita pocket bread nutritional information, see page 62

Chapatti Pocket

Servings: 4   Time: 15 minutes

Ingredients

8 Tbsp. tomato sauce
2 oz Swiss cheese, shredded
2 oz Mozzarella cheese, shredded
1/4 Cup Mushrooms, sliced
1/4 Green pepper, chopped
1/4 Red pepper, chopped
1/4 Cup onion, diced
6 Olives, sliced (green or black)

1. Pre-heat oven to 375 degrees.
2. Combine all ingredients into a medium bowl, and mix it all up.
3. Fill pockets and wrap in foil - Bake in oven for 7-8 minutes.
4. Fill pockets and serve.

Nutritional Information (per serving)

Calories	116	Cholesterol	24mg	Fiber	1g
Total Fat	8g	Sodium	416mg	Sugar	3g
Saturated Fat	4g	Carbohydrates	5g	Protein	8g

Note: For pita pocket bread nutritional information, see page 62

Appendix

- Free Foods
- Foods High in Saturated & Trans-Fats
- Vegetables Non-Starch & High Starch
- Heart Healthy Proteins
- Milk Substitutes
- Pocket Bread Equivalents
- Shopping List

Free Food List

A free food is any food or drink that contains less than 20 calories per serving. No more than 2-3 servings of these foods (with correlated portion size) should be eaten in one day, otherwise the calories of each item must be included as part of the food servings allowed in your diet plan.

Fat-Free or Reduced Fat	Serving Size
Cream cheese, fat free	1 Tbsp.
Creamers, non-dairy, liquid	1 Tbsp.
Creamers, non dairy, powder	2 tsp.
Mayonnaise fat free	1 Tbsp.
Mayonnaise, reduced fat	1 tsp.
Miracle whip, fat-free	1 Tbsp.
Miracle whip, reduced fat	1tsp.
Salad dressing, fat free or low fat	2 Tbsp.
Sour cream, fat free or reduced fat	1 Tbsp.
Non stick cooking spray	Unlimited

Sugar Free Foods	Serving Size
Jam or jelly, light	2 tsp.
Syrup, sugar free	2 Tbsp.
Candy, hard, sugar free	1 candy
Gelatin dessert, sugar free	Unlimited
Gelatin, unflavored	Unlimited
Gum, sugar free	Unlimited
Sugar substitutes	Unlimited

Liquids	Serving Size
Cocoa powder, unsweetened	1 Tbsp.
Bouillon, broth, consommé	Unlimited
Carbonated, mineral, tonic water	Unlimited
Coffee	Unlimited
Drink mixes, sugar free	Unlimited
Tea, caffeine and sugar free	Unlimited

Condiments	Serving Size
Ketchup, mustard, horseradish, relish	1 Tbsp.
Lime juice, lemon juice	1 Tbsp.
Pickle, dill (medium)	1 1/2
Salsa	1/4 cup.
Taco sauce	1 Tbsp.
Soy sauce, regular or light	1 Tbsp.
Flavoring extracts, garlic, herbs, spices	Unlimited
Tabasco, cooking wine, Worcestershire	Unlimited

Food High In Saturated & Trans-Fats

Saturated Fats: Fats found in animal products.

Meats

Goose, duck, poultry skin, giblets
Organ meat (liver, kidney)
Hot dogs, sausage or bacon

Dairy

Whole milk
Whole milk yogurt, pudding
Evaporated whole milk
High fat cheeses
Ice Cream

Fats & Oils

Lard, butter, palm oil, kernel oil, beef tallow, cocoa butter,
coconut oil, salt pork

Trans-Fats: Foods made with hydrogenated oil.
These foods typically contain hydrogenated or partially hydrogenated oil.
We recommend that you read the label.

Cake mixes, biscuit, pancake and cornbread mixes, frostings

Cakes, cookies, muffins, pies, donuts

Crackers

Peanut butter (except fresh-ground)

Frozen entrees and meals

Frozen bakery products, toaster pastries, waffles, pancakes

Most prepared frozen meats and fish (such as fish sticks)

French fries

Whipped toppings

Margarines, shortening

Instant mashed potatoes

Taco shells

Cocoa mix

Microwave popcorn

Non-starchy Vegetables

These vegetables contain high complex carbohydrates and they are loaded with nutrients and fibers. Eat these vegetables in abundance as snacks or with meals. (1 serving = 1 cup raw or 1/2 cup cooked or juiced)

Artichoke	Eggplant	Salad greens
Asparagus	Green Onions, scallions	Sauerkraut
Beans (green, wax, italian)	Kohlrabi	Spinach
Bean sprouts	Leeks	Summer squash
Beets	Mixed vegetables	Tomato, fresh
Broccoli	(without corn, peas	Turnips
Brussels Sprouts	or pasta)	Water chestnuts
Cabbage	Mushrooms	Zucchini
Carrots	Onions	
Cauliflower	Pea Pods	
Celery	Peppers (all varieties)	
Cucumber	Radishes	

Heart Healthy Proteins

- Dried beans (legumes) and peas
- Lamb: leg, loin chop, sirloin, poultry, beef tenderloin, lean beef
- Pork: tenderloin, pork loin, ham, loin chops, Canadian bacon
- Veal: loin chop, sirloin, cutlet, ground
- Venison, rabbit, buffalo, ostrich
- Reduced fat lunch meats, (less than 5 grams of fat per ounce)
- Cheese & cottage cheese (less than 3-5 grams of fat per ounce)
- Egg whites
- Tofu

Milk Substitutes

(For those who do not like milk or cannot drink it for health reasons)
1 cup of milk is equivalent to:

Yogurt, low fat, fat free	3/4 cup	Low fat frozen yogurt	1/2 cup
Cottage cheese, low fat	3/4 cup	Calcium fortified juice	3/4 cup
Low fat cheese, hard	1 1/2 ounce slice	Low fat pudding	1/2 cup
		Fortified soy milk	1 cup

Pocket Bread Equivalent

One Kangaroo Pocket is: White = 90 calories • Wheat = 80 calories

Use this as a guide when substituting any of these foods for a pocket bread.

Equivalent To	Serving Size
Traditional loaf Bread	1 slice
English muffin	1/2
Hot dog or Hamburger bun	1/2
Small Roll, plain	1
6" Tortilla (corn & flour)	1
Bran cereal	1/2 cup
Granola, low fat	1/4 cup
Grape nuts	1/4 cup
Pasta	1/3 cup
Puffed cereal	1 1/2 cups
Rice	1/3 cup
Wheat germ	3 Tbsp.
Waffle, reduced fat	1
Baked beans	1/3 cup
Corn	1/2 cup
Corn on cob	1/2 cob
Mixed veggies	1 cup
Green Peas	1/2 cup
Potato, boiled or mashed	1/2 cup
Squash, winter	1 cup
Yam, sweet potato	1/2 cup
Graham crackers	3
Popcorn, no fat	3 cups
Rice cakes	2
Saltine Crackers	6
Potato chips, baked, fat free	15-20

Shopping List

We have prepared this convenient Shopping List for you, which include most of the foods you'll need on-hand for the recipes provided in this book.

Category	Items
Meat	• Beef tenderloin, pork tenderloin • Boneless / skinless chicken breasts • Salmon & smoked, Halibut (fresh) • Imitation crab, Pre-cooked shrimp (frozen) • Sirloin tip roast & steak, Ground sirloin • Pork Loin Roast • Lean breakfast ham

ADD Your
Items to the List:

_____

_____

_____

Vegetables	• Bell peppers: red, yellow, green • Broccoli, Cabbage, Cauliflower • Cucumber, Tomato, Celery, Carrots • Onion, Scallions, Garlic, Parsley, Chives • Lettuce, Radishes, Avocado, Lemons • Alfalfa & Bean sprouts, Mushroom, Peapod • Zucchini: yellow & green

ADD Your
Items to the List:

_____

_____

_____

Fruit	• Apples, Pears • Blueberries, Raspberries, Cherries, Strawberries • Peaches, Nectarines, Oranges, Tangerines • Banana, Grapes, Kiwi • Melons, Cantaloupe

ADD Your
Items to the List:

_____

_____

_____

www.pocketdiet.com

Category	Items
Dairy	• Low fat cheeses, Feta cheese, favorites • Cream cheese (low fat, whipped) • Cottage cheese (low fat) • Yogurt, Sour cream (low fat) • Egg whites, Eggs • Fat free milk

ADD Your
Items to the List:

_____

_____

_____

Grocery / Other	• Olive oil, Canola, peanut oil, cooking spray • Tuna white albacore (in water) • Chopped walnuts, Slivered almonds, Pine nuts • Dijon Mustard, Pickle relish, Soy sauce • Low fat peanut butter, Apple jelly (low sugar) • Canned pineapple bits • Garbanzo beans (chick peas) • Fajita seasoning, ground ginger • Tahini (Sesame seed paste), Sesame seeds • Marinades: chicken, beef, pork

ADD Your
Items to the List:

_____

_____

_____

_____

_____

_____

_____

_____

Frozen	• Mixed vegetables • Hash browns, diced potatoes

ADD Your
Items to the List:

_____

_____

_____

For more information, visit:

www.pocketdiet.com

Recipes
Menu Plans
Free Newsletter
Pocket News
Downloadable ePlans
Pocket Chat
Message Board
Diet & Fitness Tips
Team Competitions
Success Stories
Pocket Buddies
Contests & Special Promotions
Shopping
Diet Support
And more...

Be sure to tell you friends and family about

The Pocket Diet!